Medical Terminology Mad

© Copyright 2024 by Publishing Help

First Edition: May 2024

Cover: Illustration made by Publishing Help

PROLOGUE

My name is Luis Alvarado, and I have been a practicing general physician for over 30 years.

This comprehensive medical terminology book is an invaluable resource for medical and nursing students entering the healthcare field.

With well-structured chapters covering foundational concepts, body systems, special senses, and advanced terminology, it provides a thorough understanding of medical language for anyone beginning their journey in this fascinating field of medicine.

The 600-question quiz incuded, ensures an excellent review and solidifies knowledge acquisition. Each chapter is meticulously organized, making complex terms accessible and easy to learn. Whether you're a student or someone just starting to work in the medical care field, this book is an essential tool for mastering medical terminology and enhancing your professional vocabulary. Highly recommended for its depth, clarity, and practical application.

I would change just one thing: the list of key terms in Chapter 8 would be more dynamic if it were divided into sections and placed at the end of each corresponding theme.

Dr. Luis Alvarado
General practitioner
Universidad Autónoma de C.A.

TABLE OF CONTENTS

PREFACE

Introduction to the Book

Welcome to Medical Terminology Made Easy, your essential learning tool for decoding complex medical jargon. As healthcare students and professionals, having a solid grasp of medical terminology is critical for effective communication and quality patient care. This book aims to demystify the intricate world of medical language so you can understand reports, diagnose conditions, and explain procedures to patients with confidence.

Medical terminology has a reputation for being intimidating and convoluted. However, at its core, it is highly organized and systematic. The key to unlocking medical vocabulary rests in understanding the component parts of medical terms: the prefixes, root words, and suffixes. When you comprehend how these fundamental pieces fit together to form words, you will be equipped to dissect and interpret all types of medical jargon.

This book will provide you with the foundation for constructing and deconstructing medical terms. We will explore the most essential prefixes, suffixes, and word roots used in clinical settings. You will learn techniques for breaking words down to analyze their meaning and usage in context. With repeated exposure and practice exercises, you will gain the skills needed to handle complex terminology with ease.

Once you have mastered the fundamentals, we will delve into terminology specific to the major body systems. You will learn about terms related to the digestive, nervous, endocrine, integumentary, and other systems. We will cover anatomy, physiology, pathological conditions, diagnostic procedures, and a wide range of clinical concepts. This knowledge will prepare you for working with patients, reading charts, and communicating with other healthcare team members.

Moving beyond physiology, you will become familiar with terminology in emerging fields such as pharmacology, genetics, oncology, and surgical innovations. We will tackle complicated clinical reports, case studies, and scenarios involving advanced medical vocabulary. You will translate terminology from theory into practical application as you build skills for the healthcare setting.

This book aims to make learning medical terminology an engaging and empowering experience. With the foundation provided here, you will have the confidence to succeed in clinical environments and nursing programs. You will gain the knowledge to play an active role in patient care discussions and excel in your education and career. Let us begin unlocking the secrets of medical language together.

Medical terminology is considered complex because medical terms consist of technical Greek and Latin roots, prefixes, and suffixes. However, the word parts follow regular patterns and rules. Once you identify the meanings of the word parts, you can break down any unfamiliar term to decipher its definition.

For instance, a basic medical term like gastroenterology is formed from the following parts:

- Gastro- = stomach
- Enter- = intestine
- -ology = study of

Put together, gastroenterology literally translates to "the study of the stomach and intestines." Knowing the meanings of the word parts allows you to decode medical terms and terminology.

First, let's review some of the most common prefixes used in medical terminology:

- a- = without
- anti- = against
- dys- = faulty, abnormal
- hyper- = excessive, over
- hypo- = under, below normal

- inter- = between
- intra- = inside
- micro- = very small
- neo- = new
- non- = absent
- pre- = before
- semi- = half
- sub- = under, moderately
- super- = excessively high

Next, we will go over the most essential suffixes in medical terminology:

- ac = pertaining to
- algia = pain
- ectomy = surgical removal
- itis = inflammation
- logist = specialist
- logy = study of
- lytic = destruction
- malacia = softening
- megaly = enlargement
- oma = tumor
- osis = diseased condition
- penia = lack of

Now that you are familiar with common prefixes and suffixes, you can start breaking down unfamiliar medical vocabulary. Let's examine the term leucopenia:

- Leuko- = white
- penia = deficiency of

Together, leucopenia translates to "a lack or deficiency of white blood cells." Practice separating other terms into their component parts to become comfortable analyzing medical terminology.

With repetition, analyzing the parts of medical terms will become second nature. You will find yourself effortlessly decoding vocabulary and using medical terminology fluently. Let's continue building your expertise by diving into anatomy, physiological conditions, and terminology specific to the major body systems.

CHAPTER 1

FOUNDATIONS OF MEDICAL TERMINOLOGY

Understanding Root Words, Prefixes, and Suffixes

To build a strong foundation in medical terminology, you must first understand the component parts of medical words: the roots, prefixes, and suffixes. Learning the meanings of these fundamental word parts allows you to break down and interpret complex vocabulary.

Word roots form the core meaning of a medical term. By recognizing a familiar root, you can get a general sense of what the word pertains to even if you have never encountered it before. Word roots are derived primarily from Greek and Latin origins. Some examples include:

- Cardio: Heart
- Neuro: Nerves
- Osteo: Bones
- Hemato: Blood
- Adeno: Glands

Let's examine the term "cardiology." By identifying the root word "cardio," you can deduce that cardiology relates to the heart. In fact, cardiology is defined as the study of the heart and its functions. Knowing that "ology" means "the study of" completes the meaning.

Prefixes can modify the meaning of a root word and provide additional context. For instance, take the prefix "hyper-" meaning excessive or overabundance and combine it with "tension" or pressure. The resulting word "hypertension" refers to abnormally high blood pressure.

Some of the most common medical prefixes you should recognize include:

- Anti-: Against
- Brady-: Slow
- Dys-: Difficulty, abnormal
- Hyper-: Excess, over
- Hypo-: Under, below normal
- Micro-: Small, tiny
- Poly-: Many
- Tachy-: Rapid, accelerated

Let's break down another example: hypotension. We take the prefix "hypo-" meaning under or below, attach it to the root "tense" for pressure, and determine hypotension means low blood pressure.

Suffixes are attached to the end of words to add nuances to the meaning of those wprds. In cardiology, for example, "-itis" denotes inflammation rather than the study of. Learning the most common suffixes enhances your ability to interpret terminology.

Examples of important suffixes in medical vocabulary include:

- algia: Pain
- ectomy: Surgical removal
- osis: Condition, disease process
- emia: Presence in blood
- logy: Study of
- tomy: Surgical incision

For instance, combining the root "arthro" meaning joint with "-itis" for inflammation creates the term "arthritis," or inflammation affecting the joints. Recognizing both components leads to an understanding of the full medical term.

Now let's try breaking down a more complex vocabulary word: gastroenterology. We can split this term into:

- Gastro-: Stomach
- Enter-: Intestine, bowel
- -ology: Study of

Combining the meanings tells us gastroenterology refers to the study of the stomach and intestines.

As you learn more word parts, you will be able to deduce the meaning of unfamiliar vocabulary by recognizing the roots, prefixes, and suffixes contained within. Developing fluency with the fundamental pieces allows you to unlock complex medical language.

It is helpful to think of word parts as reusable building blocks. By rearranging and combining them in different ways, medical professionals can assemble descriptive terminology. For example, the root "cardio" shows up in:

Electrocardiogram: Recording of heart's electrical activity

Cardiotonic: A drug that strengthens the heartbeat

Cardiomegaly: Enlargement of the heart muscle

Although long and complex, these terms share a common root that aids comprehension. Learning word parts equips you with tools to interpret endless combinations of medical vocabulary.

Let's continue building expertise in terminology by reviewing more examples:

Myocarditis combines the root "myo" for muscle, "cardio" for heart, and the suffix "-itis" denoting inflammation. Together it means inflammation of the heart muscle.

Angioplasty breaks down into "angio" referring to blood vessels, "plasty" meaning surgical repair, and the whole term signifies a procedure to widen blocked arteries.

Dyspnea contains the prefix "dys-" indicating difficult or impaired, the root "pnea" for breathing, and the full term translates to difficult or labored breathing.

Practice separating additional terms into their component parts. Try unlocking vocabulary related to oncology, pharmacology, and diagnostic procedures using your knowledge of roots, prefixes, and suffixes. With repetition, you will begin automatically recognizing word parts and fluently interpreting medical terminology. However, don't become frustrated if you cannot instantly decipher a term! Medical vocabulary encompasses a vast scope of words derived from roots, prefixes, and suffixes.

Start by mastering the most common word parts presented in this chapter. Your knowledge will steadily grow with consistent practice and exposure. Keep a running list of new roots, prefixes, and suffixes you encounter. Seeing how they combine and recombine will reinforce your learning. You now have a strong basis for tackling medical terminology by breaking words down into their fundamental parts. This will empower you to unlock the meaning of complex vocabulary and phrases throughout your medical education and career. Understanding the word parts provides you with a valuable skill set for excelling in healthcare fields.

Next, let's shift gears to discuss common terminology associated with body systems, pathological conditions, and medical interventions. We'll start with an overview of key terms related to the integumentary system of skin, hair, and nails.

The skin is the large, exterior organ that protects inner structures from damage. Medical providers need to be well-versed in integumentary system anatomy and related conditions.

Some key terms for skin anatomy include:

- Epidermis: Outer layer of skin
- Dermis: Inner skin layer containing blood vessels
- Subcutaneous: Deepest layer of fat and tissue

Common skin lesions and injuries:

- Abrasion: Area of scraped skin
- Laceration: Cut or tear in skin
- Blister: Fluid-filled skin bump
- Scar: Fibrous tissue replacing normal skin after injury

Dermatological conditions often diagnosed are:

- Eczema: Chronic inflammatory skin disorder
- Psoriasis: Autoimmune condition causing skin cell overgrowth
- Melanoma: Serious type of skin cancer
- Contact dermatitis: Rash caused by irritating or allergy-inducing substance

Treatments that specialists may perform include:

- Cryosurgery: Freezing off lesions with liquid nitrogen
- Debridement: Removal of dead or damaged skin
- Skin graft: Transplanting skin from one body part to another
- Mohs surgery: Precise surgical removal of skin cancer

With knowledge of integumentary system vocabulary, you can better understand associated pathology and treatment options. Let's continue expanding expertise by reviewing terminology related to the respiratory system next.

The respiratory system facilitates oxygen and carbon dioxide exchange through the lungs and airways. Fluency with related medical terms is vital for healthcare roles.

Key anatomical structures in the respiratory system include:

- Trachea: Windpipe connecting throat to lungs
- Bronchi: Two main airway branches entering lungs
- Alveoli: Tiny air sacs in lungs where gas exchange occurs
- Diaphragm: Major muscle aiding breathing

Common respiratory conditions include:

- Asthma: Chronic inflammation causing airway narrowing
- Pneumonia: Lung infection causing inflammation
- Emphysema: Lung damage making breathing difficult
- Pleurisy: Swelling of tissues surrounding lungs

To diagnose and treat respiratory diseases, providers may conduct:

- Spirometry: Measuring lung capacity and airflow
- Bronchoscopy: Visual examination of the airways' interior
- Thoracentesis: Draining fluid from area between chest wall and lungs
- Tracheostomy: Creating artificial airway in neck

With this review of key terminology, you are developing a strong foundation for working with respiratory disorders and treatments. Next we will focus on important vocabulary pertaining to the cardiovascular system.

Common Prefixes and Their Meanings

Prefixes play a crucial role in medical terminology, modifying meanings and providing nuance to root words and basic terms. Learning the most frequent prefixes equips you with valuable skills for deciphering vocabulary and enhancing comprehension. We will explore the most useful prefixes to know, how they consistently alter meanings, and examples terms utilizing these important word parts.

Let's begin by reviewing common prefixes indicating quantity or size:

- Uni- = One
- Mono- = One, single
- Bi- = Two
- Tri- = Three
- Quadri- = Four
- Multi- = Many
- Poly- = Many
- Hyper- = Excessive, too much
- Hypo- = Below normal, under

For example:

- Unilateral = On one side
- Mononucleosis = Condition caused by a single type of white blood cell
- Bicuspid = Two-pointed tooth
- Trigeminal = Relating to three paired nerves in the face
- Quadriplegia = Paralysis of all four limbs
- Multicystic = Containing many cysts
- Polydipsia = Excessive thirst
- Hypertension = High blood pressure
- Hypoglycemia = Low blood sugar

Learning prefixes like uni-, bi-, and poly- that indicate quantity provides helpful context and meaning for a wide range of medical terms.

Another set of useful prefixes relate to time or order:

- Primi- = First
- Pro- = Before
- Post- = After
- Neo- = New
- Chrono- = Related to time

For example:

- Primipara = Woman pregnant for the first time
- Prenatal = Existing or occurring before birth
- Postoperative = Occurring after surgery
- Neoplasm = New, abnormal growth of tissues
- Chronic = Persisting over a long period of time

Identifying temporal prefixes like pre-, post-, and chrono- enhances understanding of terminology related to timelines, sequences, and stages.

Here are other important prefixes to recognize:

- Dys- = Abnormal, difficult, impaired
- In- = Not, without

- Mal- = Poorly, bad, abnormal
- Non- = Not
- Para- = Beside, beyond
- Pseudo- = False
- Anti- = Against

For example:

- Dysphagia = Difficulty swallowing
- Insomnia = Inability to sleep
- Malignant = Cancerous, tending to metastasize
- Nontoxic = Not poisonous
- Paranoia = Irrational suspicion or fear
- Pseudoseizure = Seizure-like episode with no epileptic cause
- Antibiotic = Substance that fights infections

These prefixes consistently modify the root word to alter the overall meaning. Learning them expands your ability to interpret terminology.

Now let's discuss common prefixes used in anatomy and physiology:

- Adeno- = Gland
- Dors- = Back
- Hepato- = Liver
- Nephro- = Kidney
- Oculo- = Eye
- Pulmo- = Lung
- Vasculo- = Vessel

For example:

- Adenopathy = Disease of the glands
- Dorsalgia = Back pain
- Hepatitis = Inflammation of liver
- Nephritis = Inflammation of kidneys
- Oculorrhea = Discharge from the eye
- Pulmonology = Study of the lungs
- Vascular = Relating to blood vessels

Recognizing prefixes like nephro- and pulmo- helps identify terms related to body systems and expands anatomical/physiological vocabulary.

Next we'll cover useful prefixes related to procedures or medical specialties:

- Angio- = Vessels
- Cardi- = Heart
- Dermato- = Skin
- Endo- = Inside, within
- Onco- = Cancer, tumor
- Ortho- = Straight, correct
- Radi- = Radiation, x-rays
- Tom- = Cutting, sectioning

For example:

- Angiogram = Imaging of blood vessels

- Cardiology = Study of heart disorders
- Dermatitis = Inflammation of skin
- Endoscopy = Inserting scope inside body for examination
- Oncologist = Doctor specializing in cancer
- Orthopedics = Medical practice devoted to the skeletal system
- Radiograph = X-ray imaging
- Tomography = Cross-sectional body scanning

Learning procedure-related prefixes like angio- and cardio- builds familiarity with specialized terminology.

In summary, prefixes play a key role in medical vocabulary and systematically modifying meanings. Learning the most common prefixes allows you to interpret unfamiliar, complex terms by breaking them into recognizable parts. Mastering prefixes is crucial for enhancing comprehension and fluency in medical terminology.

Common Suffixes and Their Meanings

Along with prefixes, suffixes are fundamental components of medical vocabulary. Suffixes modify the meaning of root words and provide specificity in terminology. Learning the most useful suffixes enhances your skills for deciphering meanings and interpreting complex clinical language. We will explore some of the most common medical suffixes, how they alter the sense of base words, and example terms using these meaningful word parts.

Let's start by looking at suffixes related to anatomical concepts:

- -algia = pain
- -cele = hernia, protrusion
- -emia = presence in blood
- -gram = record or image
- -itis = inflammation
- -lysis = destruction, dissolution
- -oma = tumor, mass, swelling
- -pathy = disease
- -plasty = surgical repair

For example:

- Neuralgia = Nerve pain
- Hydrocele = Fluid-filled sac in the scrotum
- Anemia = Lack of healthy red blood cells
- Angiogram = Record of blood vessels
- Appendicitis = Inflammation of the appendix
- Thrombolysis = Breaking down blood clots
- Lipoma = Benign fatty tumor
- Cardiomyopathy = Disease of heart muscle
- Rhinoplasty = Plastic surgery of the nose

Learning suffixes like -itis and -oma provides a foundation for deciphering anatomy terminology.

Next, let's look at suffixes related to procedures:

- -centesis = surgical puncture to remove fluid
- -desis = surgical fixation
- -ectomy = excision, surgical removal
- -pexy = surgical fixation
- -plasty = surgical repair
- -rrhaphy = suturing, surgical suturing

- -stomy = creating an opening
- -tomy = incision, cutting into

For example:

Thoracentesis = Inserting a needle to drain fluid from chest cavity

- Arthrodesis = Surgically fusing a joint
- Mastectomy = Removal of the breast
- Gastropexy = Surgically attaching the stomach
- Blepharoplasty = Cosmetic eyelid surgery
- Rhinorrhaphy = Suturing the nasal septum
- Colostomy = Creating an artificial opening for the colon
- Appendectomy = Removal of the appendix

Learning procedure-based suffixes like -centesis and -tomy expands your vocabulary related to surgical interventions.

Now let's go over some suffixes related to medical specialties:

- -crine = hormone secreting glands
- -logy = study of
- -oid = resembling
- -ology = study of
- -opath = treating by means of
- -pedics = children
- -scopy = visualize, examine

For example:

- Endocrine = Relating to ductless hormone-secreting glands
- Cardiology = Study of the heart and cardiovascular system
- Carcinoid = Resembling cancer
- Psychology = Study of the mind and human behavior
- Naturopath = Physician who uses natural remedies
- Pediatrics = Branch of medicine dealing with children
- Colonoscopy = Visually examining the colon with a scope

These suffixes like -logy and -pedics help categorize and specify branches of medicine and types of treatment.

Additionally, here are some other useful suffixes to know:

- -able = capable of
- -al = relating to
- -ance = process, condition
- -ary = pertaining to
- -ic = pertaining to, characterized by
- -ion = act, process
- -ive = tending to, characterized by
- -ous = full of, containing

For example:

- Treatable = Capable of being treated
- Renal = Relating to the kidneys
- Clearance = Process of removing waste products
- Respiratory = Pertaining to respiration

- Diabetic = Characterized by diabetes
- Injection = Act of injecting into the body
- Curative = Tending to cure disease
- Fibrous = Containing or resembling fibers

These suffixes like -al, -ic, and -ous refine meanings in very helpful ways.

In summary, suffixes play a crucial role in medical terminology, systematically modifying meanings of root words. Learning common suffixes equips you with valuable skills for interpreting complex vocabulary and unfamiliar terms by recognizing meaningful word parts. Mastering the most useful suffixes will rapidly expand your fluency and comprehension.

CHAPTER 2

BODY SYSTEMS AND RELATED TERMINOLOGY

The Digestive System

Key Terms

When studying the anatomy, physiology, and pathology of the digestive system, there are many essential terms to know. Mastering key vocabulary related to the gastrointestinal tract greatly enhances comprehension of this body system. We will explore fundamental terminology pertaining to digestive organs, accessory structures, physiology, and diseases.

To begin, let's review important terms for the digestive tract organs:

Esophagus - Muscular tube connecting the throat to the stomach; transfers food from the pharynx to the stomach.

Stomach - J-shaped sac-like organ containing acid and enzymes to break down food.

Small intestine - Coiled tubular organ divided into duodenum, jejunum, and ileum segments; key site of nutrient absorption.

Large intestine - Wider, shorter tube comprised of the cecum, colon, and rectum; absorbs water from indigestible waste.

These terms for hollow organs of digestion are fundamental building blocks of gastrointestinal vocabulary.

Next, key accessory organs and structures:

Salivary glands - Produce saliva which lubricates food and contains enzymes; includes parotid, sublingual, submandibular glands.

Pancreas - Gland behind the stomach secreting enzymes for digestion and hormones to regulate blood sugar.

Gallbladder - Pear-shaped sac storing and concentrating bile from the liver.

Liver - Largest internal organ; produces bile to emulsify fats and metabolizes nutrients.

Learning terms for the salivary glands, pancreas, gallbladder and liver establishes a strong foundation for digestives system vocabulary.

Now let's discuss key physiology and processes:

Peristalsis - Rhythmic muscle contractions propelling food through the digestive tract.

Bile - Yellow-green fluid produced by the liver containing salts to emulsify fats.

Enzymes - Proteins secreted by the stomach, pancreas, and small intestine that catalyze breakdown of food.

Villi - Tiny hair-like projections in the small intestine increasing surface area for optimal absorption.

Defecation - Process of eliminating solid waste from the body through the anus.

These terms pertaining to the mechanics and functions of the GI tract are vital for comprehending digestion.

Next, terminology for common disorders:

Gastroesophageal reflux disease (GERD) - Backflow of stomach contents into the esophagus causing heartburn.

Peptic ulcer - Erosion in the lining of the stomach or duodenum.

Gallstones - Hard deposits that form in the gallbladder blocking bile flow.

Appendicitis - Inflammation of the appendix causing pain and possible rupture.

Diverticulitis - Inflamed pouches bulging out of the colon wall.

Hemorrhoids - Swollen, inflamed veins in the rectum or anus.

Knowing terms for frequent digestive diseases like GERD, ulcers, and diverticulitis enables clear communication with patients and colleagues.

Now let's reinforce this knowledge by putting the vocabulary into context:

The esophagus transports chewed food from the mouth down to the stomach by coordinated waves of muscle contractions called peristalsis. In the J-shaped stomach, food is broken down by digestive enzymes and acids. Partially digested material passes into the coiled small intestine, where bile from the gallbladder emulsifies fats, and enzymes from the pancreas continue chemical digestion. Finger-like villi lining the small intestine absorb nutrients into the bloodstream. Indigestible material travels into the large intestine for compaction and water absorption, forming feces which are then deficated through the anus, eliminating waste. Disorders like ulcers, GERD and gallstones disrupt this complex process.

This overview utilizes key terms to summarize the anatomy and function of the digestive organs. Building fluency with fundamental vocabulary lays the foundation for mastering the language of the gastrointestinal system.

The mouth, pharynx, esophagus, stomach, small intestine, large intestine, rectum and anus compose the hollow organs of the alimentary canal through which food passes during digestion. Salivary glands, pancreas, liver and gallbladder are accessory structures secreting fluids and enzymes that aid breakdown and absorption of nutrients. Specialized terms describe important anatomical structures like villi and physiological processes like peristalsis. Familiarity with terminology for common disorders such as appendicitis, GERD, and hemorrhoids enables clear communication with patients.

Learning the core vocabulary for the digestive system establishes a framework for gaining expertise with gastroenterology terminology. Combining the fundamental terms to analyze anatomy, physiology and pathology promotes deep comprehension and fluency. As you advance, continue building knowledge of word parts like *gastro-* for stomach and *-emesis* for vomiting. Integrate new terms like dysphagia, meaning difficulty swallowing, and gastritis, or inflammation of the stomach lining. Consistently reinforcing key vocabulary will steadily expand your mastery of the language of digestion.

In summary, there are essential root words, prefixes, suffixes and terminology related to the digestive system anatomy, function and disease processes. Initial focus on terms for organs like the esophagus and stomach, important physiology like enzymes and peristalsis, and common disorders such as GERD and ulcers provides a solid foundation. With regular vocabulary strengthening, you will gain skill and confidence to interpret complex gastroenterology terms by recognizing their component parts. Building expertise with the language of digestion relies on continually integrating key vocabulary into an expanding knowledge base.

Related Pathologies

The digestive system is susceptible to many disorders and diseases that can disrupt normal function, causing symptoms like abdominal pain, nausea, vomiting, and changes in bowel habits. Understanding key pathologies of the gastrointestinal tract is crucial for providing effective patient care. We will explore some of the most common digestive conditions, organized by affected organs and tissues.

Beginning with the upper digestive tract, acid reflux and GERD involve backflow of stomach contents up into the esophagus. This can lead to heartburn, irritation, and even precancerous Barrett's esophagus, if severe. Achalasia affects the lower esophageal sphincter, preventing it from properly relaxing to allow food passage. Esophagitis is inflammation of the esophageal lining, often from acid reflux. Esophageal cancers like squamous cell carcinoma can arise from repeated reflux damage.

In the stomach, gastritis refers to inflammation of the stomach lining and can be either acute or chronic. There are also peptic ulcers which are erosions in the mucosa that cause pain and bleeding, often resulting from H. pylori infection or the use of NSAIDs. Gastroparesis is another condition characterized by impaired stomach emptying due to nerve dysfunction. Pyloric stenosis involves the narrowing of the pyloric valve, leading to delayed stomach emptying. Finally, stomach cancer can manifest in various forms, such as adenocarcinoma originating from glandular cells.

The small intestine can develop inflammation and malabsorption issues. Celiac disease for instance is an autoimmune disorder where gluten damages intestinal villi, impairing nutrient absorption. Crohn's disease causes patchy inflammation anywhere in the GI tract. Short bowel syndrome is inadequate absorption due to surgical removal of small intestine. Small intestine cancers include adenocarcinoma, sarcoma, and carcinoid tumors. In the large intestine, ulcerative colitis causes diffuse inflammation and ulcers, while Crohn's disease affects patchy segments. These inflammatory bowel diseases increase colon cancer risk. Diverticulosis involves small pouches bulging from weak spots in the colon wall, which can become inflamed as diverticulitis. Irritable bowel syndrome (IBS) is abnormal contractions and sensitivity causing diarrhea/constipation. Colorectal cancers begin with polyps, becoming adenocarcinomas.

Several disorders involve the rectum and anus. Hemorrhoids are swollen, inflamed veins causing pain, bleeding, and itching. Anal fissures are small tears in the anus lining. Perianal abscesses are infected fluid collections near the anus. Anorectal fistulas are abnormal tunnels from the rectum to skin and anal cancer is typically squamous cell carcinoma.

The liver can manifest various conditions as well. Fatty liver disease ranges from steatosis to steatohepatitis and cirrhosis. Viral hepatitis involves inflammation from hepatitis virus infection. Cirrhosis causes permanent scarring and damage from various causes. Liver failure occurs when extensive damage impairs essential functions. Liver cancer includes hepatocellular carcinoma starting in liver cells. The gallbladder has several common disorders. Cholelithiasis refers to the presence of gallstones which can cause obstruction. Cholecystitis is gallbladder inflammation often due to gallstones. Gallbladder polyps are abnormal tissue growths which can become cancerous. Gallbladder cancer is most often adenocarcinoma.

Pancreatitis, or inflammation of the pancreas, can be acute or chronic. Resulting damage impairs production of enzymes and hormones like insulin. Pancreatic cancer, often starting in glandular cells, has very poor prognosis.

This overview summarizes key digestive system pathologies organized by anatomical region. Recognizing the wide range of potential conditions affecting each part of the GI tract builds clinical knowledge and informs diagnosis and treatment decisions. As you advance, continue expanding your understanding of characteristic symptoms, diagnostic approaches, risk factors and complications for each disorder. Deepening your pathology expertise will strengthen your ability to provide optimal care for patients with digestive diseases.

In diagnosing digestive conditions, the presenting symptoms provide clues to the affected regions and potential pathologies. Dysphagia and heartburn may indicate reflux or esophageal issues. Nausea and vomiting often arise from gastric pathologies like PUD or gastroparesis. Diarrhea or constipation could signify small intestine malabsorption, IBS, or inflammatory bowel disease. Rectal bleeding suggests lower GI problems like hemorrhoids, diverticulitis or colorectal cancer. Jaundice indicates liver disorders, while right upper quadrant pain suggests gallbladder disease. Knowing typical clinical presentations for digestive pathologies guides efficient, accurate diagnosis.

When evaluating digestive signs and symptoms, clinical, laboratory, and imaging tests help confirm suspected disorders. Endoscopy directly visualizes the esophagus, stomach and upper intestine, revealing inflammation, ulcers and strictures. Biopsies diagnose cancers and infections like H. pylori. Bloodwork evaluates liver function, anemia and markers of inflammation. Stool tests check for blood, bacteria, parasites and malabsorption. CT and MRI provide detailed cross-sectional abdominal imaging to assess organs, lymph nodes and tumors. Barium contrast studies visualize the digestive tract lining. Understanding appropriate diagnostic testing for suspected GI conditions optimizes accurate identification.

Treatment of digestive diseases depends on the specific pathology, severity and complications. Lifestyle changes like diet, hydration and smoking cessation support self-management of several disorders. Medications range from antacids and anti-diarrheals for symptomatic relief to antibiotics, immunosuppressants and biologics targeting underlying disease processes. Endoscopic procedures can stop bleeding ulcers, remove polyps and place feeding tubes. Surgery may be warranted for cancers, strictures, organ damage or intractable diseases. Appreciating conventional medical and surgical management of GI conditions promotes appropriate, effective care.

In summary, digestive system pathology encompasses an extensive range of potential diseases and disorders affecting the hollow organs, accessory glands and associated structures. Each region has characteristic pathological processes, from esophageal cancers to gastric ulcers to colonic polyps. Familiarity with the diverse presentations, diagnostic approaches and typical treatments for GI conditions enables knowledgeable, skillful patient care. Building expertise in digestive pathologies lays a strong foundation for clinical practice.

Diagnostic and Surgical Procedures

Evaluating and treating disorders of the digestive system often involves specialized diagnostic tests and surgical interventions. A wide array of procedures provides detailed visualization, tissue samples, access for instruments, and operative management of gastrointestinal diseases. Understanding key GI diagnostic and surgical techniques is crucial for providing appropriate patient care. We will explore some of the most important procedures for assessing and managing conditions affecting each part of the digestive tract.

Starting with the upper digestive tract, endoscopy utilizes flexible illuminated scopes inserted through the mouth to visualize the esophagus, stomach, and duodenum. This procedure can effectively diagnose various conditions such as reflux, ulcers, and cancers, and obtain biopsies if needed. Additionally, dilation during upper endoscopy can stretch narrow esophageal strictures, offering relief to patients. In cases of achalasia, peroral endoscopic myotomy (POEM) is employed to divide muscle fibers and relax the lower esophageal sphincter. Esophageal stents are utilized to open strictures, restoring proper function. For detailed imaging of the gut wall layers, upper endoscopic ultrasound (EUS) is a valuable tool. Surgical interventions, such as fundoplication, create a valve to prevent reflux, while myotomy reduces sphincter pressure in achalasia cases. Ultimately, esophagectomy may be necessary to remove cancers or severely damaged portions of the esophagus, offering patients the best chance of recovery.

For the stomach and small intestine, upper endoscopy combined with biopsy detects H. pylori infection, ulcers, gastritis, and cancers. Capsule endoscopy images the small bowel, while enteroscopy examines and treats small intestine disease using specialized endoscopes. Gastric dilation stretches narrowed pylorus, and gastrectomy surgically removes part or all of the stomach for ulcers or cancer. Small bowel resection addresses damaged segments in Crohn's disease.

Examining the large intestine and rectum, colonoscopy uses a flexible scope to visualize the colon and distal ileum. Biopsies detect inflammation, polyps and cancer. Polypectomy effectively removes precancerous polyps, reducing the risk of colorectal cancer. Lower endoscopic ultrasound offers detailed imaging of the colon and surrounding structures. Barium enema provides radiographic contrast imaging, aiding in the diagnosis of colon conditions. Colon resection is a surgical option for treating cancer, complications of diverticulitis, or severe inflammatory bowel disease. Additionally, hemorrhoid procedures are available to alleviate pain and bleeding associated with swollen tissues.

For the liver and biliary system, ultrasound provides realtime imaging of texture, lesions, and duct dilation. CT and MRI scans give detailed cross-sectional abdominal views evaluating lesions, cirrhosis and portal vein patency. Percutaneous liver biopsy samples tissue for diagnosis. Cholangiography x-ray images the bile ducts after contrast injection. ERCP combines endoscopy and contrast to image the pancreatic and bile ducts, obtain cytology, and remove stones. Cholecystectomy laparoscopically removes the gallbladder for stones or cancer.

The pancreas can be evaluated by CT, MRI, ultrasound, and endoscopic ultrasound to examine tissues and ducts for masses, cysts or stones. Endoscopic retrograde cholangiopancreatography (ERCP) images the pancreatic duct. Biopsy samples cells for diagnosis and pancreatectomy removes pancreatic malignancies and head of pancreas masses compressing bile ducts.

This overview describes major diagnostic and surgical GI procedures, stressing indications and techniques for key tests and operations in managing various digestive disorders. Advancing your familiarity with how endoscopy, imaging, biopsies and resection surgeries are utilized will strengthen your capacity to make appropriate procedural recommendations and referrals for optimal patient care.

When evaluating digestive signs and symptoms, selecting the right procedures relies on diagnostic reasoning correlating clinical presentation with suspected anatomical regions and pathologies. Dysphagia suggests upper endoscopy to examine the esophagus. Persistent heartburn warrants endoscopy to assess for GERD complications like esophagitis, strictures, Barrett's esophagus. Abdominal pain and diarrhea indicates colonoscopy to evaluate for IBD. Jaundice and right upper quadrant pain prompts ultrasound and potentially ERCP to examine the biliary system. Combining knowledge of GI pathologies and procedure capabilities guides effective, efficient diagnosis.

It is important to note that the risks and benefits of diagnostic tests should be considered when formulating procedural plans. Endoscopy risks include perforation and bleeding, increased in therapeutic interventions like polypectomy. Radiation exposure from CT scans raises lifetime cancer risk. Sedation required for endoscopy and anesthesia for surgery have cardiopulmonary side effects. Balancing procedural risks against the value of diagnostic information is key for patient-centered care.

Incorporating diagnostic findings, pathology results, patient preferences and surgical expertise determines optimal treatment plans. Early cancers found by endoscopy may be cured by endoscopic resection or limited surgery while advanced cancers require radical resection. Gastroparesis refractory to medication may warrant gastric pacemaker placement. Intractable ulcerative colitis not responding to maximal medical therapy may necessitate colectomy. Multidisciplinary input choosing the least invasive options with the best outcomes is ideal.

In summary, specialized procedures enable thorough assessment and tailored treatment of digestive diseases. Strategic selection of endoscopy, imaging, biopsy and surgical techniques requires in-depth understanding of pathologies, procedural capabilities, risks and benefits. Combining procedural expertise with diagnostic acumen and collaboration yields customized management maximizing benefit while minimizing harm. Mastering use of key GI diagnostic and surgical modalities is crucial for optimal patient care.

The Cardiovascular System

Key Terms

The cardiovascular system encompasses the heart, an intricate network of blood vessels, and the circulating blood itself. Learning anatomy and physiology related terminology provides a foundation for understanding normal cardiac structure and function, common diseases, and clinical assessments. We will explore fundamental vocabulary for cardiovascular structures, processes, and pathologies.

Beginning with basic cardiac anatomy, it is crucial to know terms referring to chambers, valves, vessels, and electrical conduction:

Atria - The upper receiving chambers of the heart.

Ventricles - Lower pumping chambers of the heart.

Tricuspid and mitral valves - Regulate blood flow into the ventricles.

Aortic and pulmonic valves - Regulate blood exiting the ventricles.

Coronary arteries - Supply oxygenated blood to the heart muscle.

Cardiac veins - Drain deoxygenated blood from the heart.

Sinoatrial and atrioventricular nodes - Generate electrical impulses.

Learning the names and functions of these key cardiac structures establishes a framework for building cardiovascular knowledge.

Understanding how the heart functions as a pump relies on comprehending physiological processes and cycles:

Cardiac output - Volume of blood pumped by the heart per minute.

Stroke volume - Blood ejected per ventricular contraction.

Heart rate - Number of heart beats per minute.

Systole - Ventricular contraction phase of heart cycle.

Diastole - Ventricular relaxation phase of the cycle.

Cardiac cycle - All events in one heartbeat.

Fluency with these fundamental terms facilitates deeper comprehension of hemodynamics.

Next, key vocabulary pertaining to the vascular system:

Arteries - Vessels carrying blood away from the heart.

Veins - Vessels returning blood to the heart.

Capillaries - Microscopic vessels exchanging with tissues.

Endothelium - Cell layer lining vessel interiors.

Smooth muscle - Controls vessel diameter.

These vascular anatomy basics provide building blocks for understanding circulation.

Now, essential terminology related to common cardiac disorders:

Atherosclerosis - Plaque accumulation in artery walls.

Ischemia - Inadequate blood supply to tissues.

Infarction - Tissue death from blocked blood flow.

Arrhythmia - Abnormal heart rhythm.

Aneurysm - Ballooning weak spot in a blood vessel.

Hypertension - Abnormally high blood pressure.

Heart failure - Impaired cardiac pumping function.

Familiarity with terms for frequent cardiovascular diseases facilitates clear communication with patients.

Let's connect this vocabulary to cardiac physiology concepts:

Oxygenated blood returning from the lungs fills the left atrium during diastole. As the atria contract, blood flows into the ventricles through the open mitral and tricuspid valves. Ventricular contraction in systole forces blood out through the aortic and pulmonic valves, generating stroke volume and cardiac output. Coronary arteries deliver oxygen and nutrients to the actively contracting heart muscle. Multiplying the stroke volume by the heart rate determines cardiac output.

Integrating key terms reinforces comprehension of normal cardiovascular function. Building fluency with essential vocabulary lays a strong foundation for learning the language of cardiology.

In summary, there are many important root words, prefixes, suffixes and terminology related to cardiac anatomy, vascular structures, hemodynamics, and common diseases. Initial focus on fundamentals like chambers, valves, arteries and veins establishes a framework for constructing cardiovascular vocabulary knowledge. Regularly strengthening this language base by studying new cardiology terms in the context of core concepts will steadily enhance expertise and confidence. Consistent review of key vocabulary is vital for mastery of the intricate language of the cardiovascular system.

Related Pathologies

The cardiovascular system is susceptible to many disorders that can disrupt normal heart function and blood circulation. Gaining familiarity with common cardiac and vascular diseases is key for providing effective evaluation and management of patients. We will explore some of the most prevalent cardiovascular pathologies.

Beginning with the heart, coronary artery disease develops as fatty plaque accumulates in vessel walls, causing narrowing called stenosis. This reduces blood supply to heart muscle, resulting in ischemia, arrhythmias, and myocardial infarction if severe. Heart valve disorders like mitral valve prolapse and aortic stenosis disturb normal blood flow. Cardiomyopathies affect the heart muscle itself, often leading to enlargement and impaired pumping. Congestive heart failure results when the weakened heart cannot meet metabolic demands.

Arrhythmias arise from electrical abnormalities causing irregular heart rates and rhythms. Tachycardias involve excessively rapid firing, while bradycardias are slow heart rates. Atrial fibrillation produces irregular quivering of the upper chambers. Ventricular fibrillation causes chaotic activity that causes cardiac arrests if not corrected. Heart blocks interrupt normal conduction between upper and lower chambers.

Moving to the vascular system, it's important to note that atherosclerosis can impact any artery in the body. Plaque buildup in the carotid artery poses a significant risk for stroke, renal artery stenosis can lead to hypertension and peripheral arterial disease restricts blood supply to the limbs, resulting in claudication pain. Aortic aneurysms are weakened bulges in the aorta that may rupture, causing potentially fatal bleeding. Varicose veins are twisted, enlarged superficial veins that commonly cause leg swelling and pain.

Hypertension, or chronically elevated blood pressure, increases incidence of atherosclerosis, heart failure, kidney disease and stroke if prolonged. Elevated cholesterol levels directly accelerate atheroma formation in vessel walls. Diabetes mellitus disturbs fat and glucose metabolism, promoting accelerated cardiovascular disease.

Thromboembolic disease involves clot formation obstructing blood flow. Deep vein thrombosis leads to pulmonary embolism that can result in right heart strain and death. Myocardial infarction and many strokes stem from clots blocking coronary or cerebral arteries. Anticoagulant medication therapy reduces the clotting risk in susceptible individuals.

In summary, the cardiovascular system is afflicted by numerous pathologies affecting the heart, vessels and circulation. Coronary disease and heart failure compromise muscle function. Rhythm disturbances disrupt effective pumping. Atherosclerosis and hypertension multiply complications across organs. Clots produce abrupt ischemia. Recognizing typical presentations facilitates accurate diagnosis and management. Further deepening pathology knowledge better equips providers to optimize care for the many patients experiencing cardiac and vascular disease.

Optimal evaluation and treatment of cardiovascular pathologies relies on correlation between presentation and suspected disorder. Chest pain, shortness of breath, arrhythmias or syncope prompt workup for coronary ischemia, heart failure and conduction abnormalities. Stroke or TIA symptoms warrant imaging to identify emboli, thrombi or vessel stenosis. Hypertension guidelines direct individualized medication regimens. Anticoagulation for atrial fibrillation, heart failure or post-thrombotic states balances thromboembolism risk against bleeding odds. Tailoring management to address the most likely underlying pathology improves outcomes.

Cardiovascular diagnosis requires selection of suitable testing modalities based on clinical context. The ECG provides baseline cardiac rhythm and hypertrophy evidence. Cardiac enzymes diagnose myocardial infarction. Stress testing assesses coronary ischemia. Echocardiography defines chamber size, wall motion and valve structure and motion. MRI quantifies ventricular function and viability. CT angiography delineates coronary stenosis. It is important to understanding the appropriate use of specific tests as this ensures efficient diagnosis.

The treatment of these pathologies integrates lifestyle modification, medications, device therapies and procedures. Smoking cessation, blood pressure control, glucose and lipid regulation, and anticoagulation for stroke risk all mitigate cardiovascular disease progression. Medications encompass beta blockers, ACE inhibitors, statins and antiplatelet agents. Implantable pacemakers and defibrillators correct arrhythmias. Stenting expands narrowed arteries. Heart valve repair or replacement surgery restores function. Carefully tailored management optimizes outcomes for each patient's condition.

In summary, cardiovascular pathology spans a spectrum ranging from conduit vessel disease to structural heart disorders to circulatory deficits. Fluent familiarity with common presentations, workup modalities, and therapeutic management of cardiac and vascular pathologies provides the foundation for excellence in patient care. Steadily building expertise in this complex domain is key for practicing proficient cardiology.

Diagnostic and Surgical Procedures

Assessing and treating cardiovascular disorders relies heavily on specialized diagnostic tests and surgical interventions. Mastering current modalities for imaging, monitoring, sampling, and operating on the heart and vessels is fundamental for providing optimal patient care. We will explore some of the most important cardiovascular procedures.

Beginning with diagnosis, electrocardiography (ECG) records the heart's electrical activity, detecting arrhythmias and ischemia. Echocardiography uses ultrasound to evaluate chamber size, wall motion, valve function and pulmonary pressures. Stress echocardiography assesses function during induced ischemia. Cardiac CT angiography visualizes coronary artery stenosis. MRI precisely quantifies ventricular volumes, function and viability without radiation. Catheterization measures chamber pressures and oxygen saturation while angiography images vessels.

Ambulatory ECG monitoring tools include Holter monitors recording 24+ hour rhythms and event recorders activated by patients when symptomatic. Implantable loop recorders continually monitor rhythms for years, automatically activating to capture arrhythmias. Cardiac stress testing induces controlled ischemia to reveal functional limits. Exercise stress ECG monitors for ST segment changes indicating ischemia. Pharmacologic stress echocardiography or nuclear imaging add imaging evidence of ischemia or infarcts.

Examining blood provides valuable insights into cardiovascular health. Complete blood counts help identify anemia, which can reduce oxygen delivery throughout the body. Cardiac enzymes, such as troponin, play a crucial role in diagnosing myocardial infarction. Natriuretic peptides offer predictive information regarding the risk of heart failure. Lipid panels reveal risk factors for atherosclerosis and coagulation studies help guide dosing for anticoagulant therapy. Tissue samples further define cardiac disorders. Cardiac catheterization enables myocardial biopsy evaluating infiltrative diseases. Vascular biopsy assesses vessel inflammation and cholesterol content. Providing enough diagnostic information guides management.

Interventional cardiology deploys catheter-based tools to treat vascular and structural heart disease. Angioplasty balloons widen narrowed arteries while stents scaffold them open. Catheter ablation destroys aberrant conduction pathways causing arrhythmias. Percutaneous valve procedures involve implanting new valves within diseased ones, while septal defect closure devices are used to patch abnormal openings. It's crucial to understand the capabilities and limitations of these catheter interventions.

Cardiac surgery addresses complex structural disorders and advanced coronary disease. Coronary artery bypass grafting involves implanting vessels to bypass blockages. Valve repair or replacement is used to treat severe stenosis and regurgitation. Maze procedures are performed to ablate arrhythmia substrates. Ventricular assist devices are utilized to support profound heart failure as bridges to transplant. Familiarity with the indications and techniques for these procedures is essential in guiding surgery referrals.

Endovascular surgery uses wire-guided tools navigated from within blood vessels. Aortic aneurysm stent grafts reinforce dangerously enlarged sections, while carotid artery stenting stabilizes vulnerable atherosclerotic plaque. Renal artery stenting improves blood flow to ischemic kidneys. Understanding vascular surgery options is valuable.

This overview describes the major modalities for diagnosing and treating cardiovascular diseases. Advancing expertise with stress testing, imaging, catheterization, multimodality monitoring, and the range of surgical interventions will strengthen capacity to provide prompt, effective cardiovascular care. The extensive cardiology procedural repertoire demands dedication to continual learning.

In summary, mastering appropriate use of diagnostic testing, interventional procedures, and cardiovascular surgery is central to high quality patient care. Combining procedural knowledge with clinical acumen allows for the optimization of tailored management plans, aligning options with individual risks and benefits. Dedication to regularly expanding procedural skills and utilizing new modalities enables the delivery of the most advanced cardiovascular care.

The Respiratory System

Key Terms

The respiratory system facilitates gas exchange between the environment and bloodstream through breathing. Building a robust vocabulary equips us to clearly discuss anatomy, physiology, diagnosis and disease related to this vital system. We will explore fundamental terminology underpinning respiratory medicine.

Starting with upper airway structures, key terms include:

Nose - External protrusion warming and humidifying air.

Nasal cavity - Interior nasal passage lined with mucosa.

Pharynx - Throat region behind nose and mouth.

Larynx - Voice box containing vocal cords.

Knowing the names and functions of these upper structures establishes an anatomical foundation.

Moving lower in the tract:

Trachea - Windpipe conducting air to lungs.

Bronchi - Branches from trachea entering lungs.

Bronchioles - Narrower airway branches within lungs.

Alveoli - Microscopic air sacs transferring gases.

Fluency with these central airway terms enables conceptualizing flow.

Understanding ventilation requires breathing phase vocabulary:

Inspiration - Inhalation bringing air into lungs.

Expiration - Exhalation expelling air.

Tidal volume - Air inhaled or exhaled in one breath.

Minute ventilation - Tidal volume multiplied by rate.

These measurements quantify central respiratory parameters.

Gas exchange relies on pressure gradients:

Partial pressure - Proportion of total gas pressure exerted by one component.

Alveolar and arterial oxygen pressures - O2 pressures in alveoli and arteries.

Ventilation/perfusion ratio - Matching of air reaching and blood passing alveoli.

Grasp of these concepts empowers discussing oxygenation.

Diagnostic testing terminology includes:

Spirometry - Measuring inhalation and exhalation air volumes.

Peak flow - Maximum exhalation speed.

Pulse oximetry - Estimating arterial blood oxygen saturation.

ABG - Arterial blood gas assessing oxygen and carbon dioxide pressures.

Imaging - Xrays, CT scans and MRIs visualizing structures.

Knowing these techniques facilitates recommending appropriate studies.

Finally, pathology vocabulary:

COPD - Chronic obstructive pulmonary disease like emphysema.

Asthma - Periodic airway narrowing and bronchospasm.

Pneumonia - Lung infection causing inflammation.

Pulmonary edema - Fluid accumulation in airspaces.

Pulmonary embolism - Lodged clot blocking arterial blood flow.

Comprehending disease terms enables productive discussions.

Integrating this foundational vocabulary lays the groundwork for learning respiratory medicine language. Studying the meaning and usage of key terms provides building blocks to articulate anatomy, physiology, evaluation and pathology concepts clearly and accurately. Respiratory fluency empowers improving care through precise communication.

In summary, mastering fundamental respiratory terminology like airway anatomy, ventilation metrics, gas exchange principles, diagnostic modalities and common diseases establishes a firm footing for expanding expertise. Regular vocabulary strengthening exercises utilizing core concepts in context will steadily enhance comprehension and confidence. Consistent review cementing your grasp of essential respiratory words and phrases is the surest path to mastery of this intricate technical language underpinning the field.

Related Pathologies

The respiratory system faces threats from infectious insults, inflammatory conditions, obstructive diseases and neoplastic disorders. Building familiarity with common pulmonary pathologies is key for providing prompt, effective diagnosis and management. We will explore some prevalent respiratory diseases.

Beginning with infections, pneumonia arises when bacteria, viruses or fungi reach the alveoli, eliciting inflammation and fluid accumulation. Symptoms of fever, cough, dyspnea and chest pain along with imaging findings direct appropriate antibiotic therapy. Tuberculosis, a serious bacterial pneumonia, requires prolonged multidrug treatment. Fungal pneumonia frequently strikes immunocompromised patients.

Chronic obstructive pulmonary disease (COPD) encompasses emphysema, which destroys alveolar walls, and chronic bronchitis inflames and scars airways. Cigarette smoking is the major risk factor. Shortness of breath, wheezing, cough and reduced exercise tolerance, signal COPD's progressive airflow limitation. Treatment may include smoking cessation, bronchodilators, steroids and oxygen for advanced disease.

Asthma features episodic airway constriction, bronchospasm and excessive mucus production, often triggered by allergens or irritants. Wheezing, coughing, and chest tightness during exacerbations respond to bronchodilators and anti-inflammatory agents. Long-term control aims to prevent attacks through trigger avoidance, medications and monitoring airflow obstruction.

Pulmonary embolism occurs when clots travel to the lungs, lodging in arteries and abruptly blocking blood flow. Symptoms like chest pain and shortness of breath combined with risk factors prompt diagnostic workup to direct anticoagulant therapy preventing further embolization.

Lung cancer often arises from airway epithelial cells damaged by carcinogen exposure. Local effects like cough, dyspnea and bleeding combine with systemic symptoms as tumors spread. Lung cancer screening aims to detect early stage disease when surgical resection provides best outcomes.

Interstitial lung disease covers a heterogeneous group of disorders causing progressive scarring of lung tissue. Presentations involve dyspnea, cough and reduced capacity. Treatment centers on immuno-suppressive medications to slow decline. Idiopathic pulmonary fibrosis is a common interstitial lung disease without a confirmed cause.

Building expertise in recognizing typical presentations of prevalent respiratory pathologies enables prompt, effective management protecting lung function. Further deepening knowledge of pulmonary medicine better equips providers to optimize care for the many patients experiencing respiratory disease.

Careful history taking and physical examination focusing on respiratory signs and symptoms, guide appropriate selection of diagnostic studies. Imaging like chest Xrays and CT scans define lung anatomy, infection, masses and interstitial changes. Spirometry quantifies airflow limitations assisting COPD diagnosis and asthma monitoring. Pulse oximetry reveals hypoxemia indicating potential pneumonia or pulmonary embolism. Bloodwork can identify infection or inflammation. Specialized testing like bronchoscopy with biopsy provides definitive tissue diagnosis when needed.

Respiratory disease management integrates pharmacotherapy, devices, rehab and procedures. Inhaled bronchodilators and steroids alleviate airway constriction in COPD and asthma. Antibiotics treat pneumonia. Anticoagulants prevent pulmonary embolism recurrence. Chemotherapy, radiation and surgery aim to cure lung cancer when possible. Oxygen supports hypoxemic patients. Pulmonary rehabilitation builds exercise tolerance. Thoughtfully tailored, evidence-based care optimizes outcomes.

In summary, respiratory pathology ranges from infections to airflow limitations to malignancies. Recognition of typical disease presentations, knowledge of diagnostic options, and fluency in therapeutic management equip providers to improve care. Dedication to continuously expanding expertise across the breadth of pulmonary medicine best positions one to address diverse respiratory problems.

Diagnostic Techniques

Assessing respiratory status and disease relies on various diagnostic tests evaluating anatomy, function, and physiology. Developing proficiency interpreting key studies facilitates accurate diagnosis and tailored management. We will explore essential respiratory diagnostic modalities and techniques.

A chest x-ray produces a two-dimensional image of lung anatomy highlighting abnormalities like masses, pneumonias, and pleural effusions. While useful as an initial study, x-ray lacks sensitivity for subtle or diffuse processes. CT scanning provides 3D views and better defines lung structural detail and lesions but with higher radiation exposure.

Spirometry measures airflow parameters such as forced vital capacity (FVC), forced expiratory volume (FEV), and FEV/FVC ratio. Reduced measurements indicate obstructive or restrictive pathology. Regular spirometry monitoring aids asthma and COPD assessment. Peak expiratory flow (PEF) monitors max exhalation speed and is useful for asthma self-management.

Pulse oximetry estimates arterial oxygen saturation and screening for hypoxemia. ABG directly measures arterial oxygen and carbon dioxide partial pressures, acid-base status and oxygen content, which helps to determine if respiratory failure is present.

Exhaled nitric oxide testing assesses airway inflammation, which is useful for asthma management. 6-minute walk testing evaluates exercise capacity and oxygenation. Cardiopulmonary exercise testing provides detailed cardio-respiratory response data during exertion up to maximal effort.

Bronchoscopy allows visual inspection of airways and collection of samples like bronchial washings, brushings and biopsies. Endobronchial ultrasound aids lymph node and mass sampling. Bronchoalveolar lavage samples alveoli, useful in pneumonia and interstitial lung disease.

Sleep studies monitor overnight respiration detecting disorders like obstructive sleep apnea. Pulmonary function tests measure lung volumes like vital capacity and functional residual capacity, gauging restrictive defects. Diffusing capacity quantifies gas exchange efficiency and is reduced in emphysema.

Chest imaging, spirometry, oximetry, blood gas analysis and bronchoscopy comprise the core diagnostic techniques for assessing most respiratory disorders. Additional specialized modalities provide complementary physiological details. Understanding the optimal tests for evaluating common symptoms and diseases is key.

In summary, mastering appropriate application of the diverse respiratory diagnostic studies facilitates accurate diagnosis, integrated with clinical presentation. Thoughtfully selecting the proper modalities avoids unnecessary testing and radiation. Developing strong interpretive skills builds capacity to guide management with testing outcomes rather than testing alone.

Additional critical diagnostic skills include correctly obtaining quality sputum samples for culture and microscopy when pneumonia is suspected. Recognizing when more invasive sampling like bronchoscopy is truly needed, prevents unnecessary procedures. Providing clear pre-test education ensures optimal patient effort for valid spirometry and exercise study results. Careful review of spirometry traces avoids over-interpretation of variations within normal range. Competent at peak flow instruction ensures patients obtain useful home monitoring data. Knowledgeably advising on sleep study preparation increases diagnostic yield. Preventing inadequate or excessive testing through solid understanding of optimal modalities improves care, outcomes and costs.

Fluency with respiratory diagnostic techniques comes with regular hands-on practice. Seeking opportunities to apply various modalities across diverse patient scenarios cements understanding of the optimal role each plays. Gaining direct experience with spirometry enhances recognition of technical errors and submaximal effort affecting results. Reviewing numerous ABGs sharpens interpretation skills, readily recognizing primary derangements versus compensation. Observing sleep studies teaches nuances like differentiating central from obstructive apnea. Immersive learning builds lasting expertise.

The Nervous System

Key Terms

The nervous system controls and integrates all functions of the human body through networks transmitting electrochemical signals. Mastering the extensive terminology underlying nervous system anatomy, physiology, disease and treatment establishes a critical foundation for learning. We will explore key nervous system vocabulary essential for discussing this intricate body system.

The central nervous system contains the brain and spinal cord. The brain has regions like the cerebrum, cerebellum and brainstem, each with distinct roles. The spinal cord carries the signals between body and brain.

The peripheral nervous system contains the somatic, autonomic and enteric components. The somatic system transmits sensations and signals to skeletal muscles. The autonomic system regulates involuntary functions through sympathetic and parasympathetic divisions. The enteric system controls the gastrointestinal tract.

Neurons are electrically excitable cells transmitting signals through specialized connections called synapses. Supporting glial cells nourish, insulate and protect these neurons. Action potentials are brief electrical impulses propagating along neurons and neurotransmitters are chemicals that neurons release to communicate across synapses.

Key brain anatomy terminology includes lobes like frontal, parietal, temporal and occipital. Convoluted surface features such as sulci and gyri, and deep structures like the basal ganglia, hippocampus and amygdala. Understanding spinal cord tracts like the corticospinal and spinothalamic facilitates discussing symptoms.

Knowing receptor types like nociceptors sensing pain, proprioceptors detecting body position and chemoreceptors activated by specific substances enables explaining sensory detection. Mastering effector categories including exocrine glands secreting substances and effector organs like cardiac and smooth muscle empowers discussing responses.

Grasping neurophysiology requires terms like resting potential, threshold, synaptic transmission, neural integration and neural plasticity. Fluency with the blood brain barrier, cerebrospinal fluid and meninges strengthens discussions of central nervous system physiology.

Neurological disease vocabulary include stroke, seizures, dementia, movement disorders, neuromuscular diseases, infectious diseases, headaches, spine disorders and brain tumors. Psychiatry terminology covers disorders like depression, anxiety, psychosis and addiction. Understanding treatments requires knowing terms like neuropharmacology, neurosurgery, radiosurgery and rehabilitation.

In summary, the expansive nervous system lexicon can seem daunting. Regularly strengthening vocabulary knowledge through review, testing and usage in context, cements mastery of essential terminology, enhancing learning capacity. Deep familiarity with core concepts empowers fluent discussion of nervous system structure, function and disorders.

Common Disorders

The nervous system is susceptible to many diseases and injuries causing devastating impacts on sensation, movement, cognition, emotion and more. Building expertise in recognizing, diagnosing and managing prevalent neurological disorders is critical for effective care. We will survey some of the major categories of nervous system pathology.

Cerebrovascular disease encompasses strokes, where vessels supplying the brain are occluded by thrombi or rupture. Ischemic strokes cause focal deficits like hemiparesis, reflecting localized brain injury. Hemorrhagic strokes induce diffuse symptoms including headache and altered consciousness. Rapid stroke treatment aims to restore blood flow and prevent further damage.

Seizures arise from abnormal electrical discharges in the brain, manifesting in behaviors like convulsions or staring spells depending on the affected region. Epilepsy causes recurrent unprovoked seizures, treated with anticonvulsants and sometimes surgery. Distinguishing syncope, a loss of consciousness from reduced blood flow, is vital to avoid misdiagnosis.

Neurodegenerative diseases progressively damage neurons, impairing movement and cognition. Alzheimer's disease involves amyloid plaques and neuronal dysfunction inducing memory loss and confusion. Parkinson's disease features tremor, stiffness and slowed movement from basal ganglia degeneration. No cures currently exist, so optimizing quality of life is the focus.

Demyelinating disorders damage the myelin insulating axons, disrupting signal conduction. Multiple sclerosis causes episodes of visual loss, weakness and incoordination corresponding to areas of myelin breakdown. Supportive care aims to manage symptoms and slow progression.

Neuromuscular diseases impair communication at the neuromuscular junction, weakening the muscles. Myasthenia gravis provokes fatigable weakness. Effective treatments include cholinesterase inhibitors and immunosuppression. Muscular dystrophies cause progressive wasting from genetic defects affecting muscle proteins. Physical therapy helps maintain function.

Headaches arise from irritation of pain-sensitive head structures. Migraines induce severe unilateral pain with light and sound sensitivity. Cluster headaches cause excruciating unilateral pain in clusters. Treatments range from pain relievers to preventive medications. Identifying secondary causes like hemorrhage requires prompt neuroimaging.

Movement disorders affect control of voluntary and involuntary motions. Parkinson's disease causes slowness, rigidity and tremor from basal ganglia dysfunction. Essential tremor prompts shaking during intentional movement. Pharmacotherapy, physical therapy and sometimes surgery provide symptom relief.

Spine disorders impinge on the spinal cord and nerve roots, causing pain, weakness and numbness in affected areas. Herniated discs compress nerve roots, typically improving with conservative care. Spinal stenosis narrows the central canal, requiring surgical decompression in serious cases.

In summary, this overview highlights some major nervous system disorder categories. Recognizing characteristic presentations guides appropriate workup and treatment. Continuously strengthening core knowledge better equips providers to improve care across this broad spectrum of neurologic disease.

Effective management integrates thorough history taking, detailed neurological examination, and supporting diagnostic studies. Key historical factors include onset, course, exacerbating and alleviating factors, associated symptoms, and family history of neurological disease. Examination documents vital signs, mental status, cranial nerves, motor function, reflexes, sensation and coordination. Brain imaging like CT and MRI detects structural lesions. Spinal imaging can reveal disc and canal pathology. Electroencephalography records electrical discharges in seizures and encephalopathy. Electromyography evaluates neuromuscular transmission and muscle health. Cerebrospinal fluid analysis aids diagnosis of infections and inflammatory disorders.

Pharmacotherapy addresses many neurological issues. Anticonvulsants treat seizures, neurotransmitter modulators improve Parkinson's symptoms, disease modifying agents slow multiple sclerosis progression and analgesics relieve headaches. Physical, occupational and speech therapy boost functional capacity while surgery is warranted for amenable tumors, vascular malformations and some movement disorders.

Integrating clinical findings with appropriate diagnostic testing distinguishes neurological mimics, guides treatment, and monitors progression. Keeping current with evolving diagnostic and therapeutic technologies enables optimizing care.

Treatment and Management

Nervous system disorders encompass a vast array of diseases and injuries affecting the brain, spinal cord, nerves and muscles. Optimizing patient outcomes relies on prompt, accurate diagnosis guiding appropriate therapeutic interventions to alleviate symptoms and limit disability. We will explore key elements of managing common neurological conditions.

The first priority in acute neurological settings like possible stroke or seizure is stabilizing the patient through measures including airway protection, supplemental oxygen, cardiac monitoring and correcting unstable vital signs. Preventing further neural injury remains paramount before definitive diagnosis. Emergent cases may require neuroimaging, lumbar puncture or EEG depending on presentations.

Chronic management hinges on accurate diagnosis based on thorough history, physical examination and selection of appropriate tests. Distinguishing neurological mimics like migraine versus mass lesion headache directs proper therapy. Updated imaging and cerebrospinal fluid analysis often assist diagnosis. Electrodiagnostic studies support localizing nerve injuries. Pharmacotherapy forms the mainstay for many neurological diseases. Anti-epileptic drugs prevent seizures by reducing excitability and neural firing. Parkinson's medications replace dopamine, inhibit acetylcholine or stimulate dopamine receptors to improve movement. Immunomodulating agents slow multiple sclerosis progression by blunting inflammation. Promptly identifying and addressing medication side effects improves compliance.

Neurorehabilitation maximizes function in disorders causing impairment. Physical, occupational and speech therapy help patients adapt to disabilities using compensatory techniques and assistive devices. Counseling provides psychosocial support for coping and vocational rehabilitation enables returning to work appropriately. The introduction of Early rehabilitation intervention produces optimal gains. Surgical interventions treat amenable conditions unresponsive to conservative therapy. Examples include tumor resection, draining intracranial hematomas causing mass effect, revascularization for ischemic disease, deep brain stimulation for movement disorders, nerve decompression and disentangling neural tissue. Thorough discussion of the risks and benefits ensures appropriate procedures. Supportive critical care often maintains function until deficits resolve or definitive treatment options become available. Airway management, mechanical ventilation, intracranial pressure monitoring, sedation protocols and controlling secondary injury prevents losing ground. Multimodal monitoring guides treatment of unstable patients. Palliative approaches maximize comfort at life's end for disorders lacking curative therapies. There is also, compassionate end-of-life discussion, which ensures aligning care with patient values and goals. Hospice provides holistic interdisciplinary support as decline progresses.

In summary, optimizing neurological care requires promptly matching appropriate therapies to accurate diagnoses to limit suffering and disability. This necessitates continuously cultivating expertise across the full spectrum of neurological conditions and management options. Critical knowledge for effective management includes typical disease trajectories, expected responses to interventions, recognizing complications, and navigating sometimes narrow therapeutic windows.

For example, Parkinson's medications require meticulous titration and timing to balance symptom control and side effects like dyskinesia. Multiple sclerosis treatment choices depend on disease course, with very active relapsing-remitting disease warranting stronger immunotherapy. Post-stroke rehabilitation strives for early mobility to maximize cerebral plasticity while avoiding overexertion raising intracranial pressure. Such nuanced understanding guides tailoring therapy to each patient's unique disease profile and evolving status. It requires dedicated self-directed learning through practice experience, mentors, and consulting evidence-based guidelines. Attending professional conferences exposes clinicians to the latest therapeutic advances.

Mindfully integrating new technologies like robotic assistive devices and genomic medicine into practice optimizes utilizing exciting innovations. However, unproven interventions should be avoided until validated through rigorous study. A balanced approach thoughtfully applies promising developments backed by early evidence, while ensuring traditional basics remain the foundation.

CHAPTER 3

SPECIAL SENSES AND RELATED MEDICAL TERMS

The Visual System

Anatomy and Key Terms

Vision facilitates interacting with the surrounding environment by converting light into neural signals interpreted by the brain. The intricate structures mediating visual perception each contribute unique functions. We will survey core visual apparatus anatomy and key terminology underlying sight.

Beginning at the surface, the cornea and lens focus entering light onto the retina lining the posterior chamber. The iris adjusts light levels by dilating and constricting the pupil aperture. Lacrimal glands produce tear film moisturizing the ocular surface. The retina houses photoreceptor cells transducing light into electrical signals conveyed by retinal ganglion cells forming the optic nerve. Cones support color vision concentrated in the fovea centralis. Rods distributed peripherally enable night vision. Supporting cells nourish and interconnect neurons. Visual information is processed by distinct parallel pathways. The magnocellular pathway mediates motion perception and eye movements via rapid signal transmission. The parvocellular pathway enables detailed conscious visual perception by projecting to the lateral geniculate nucleus and then primary visual cortex.

Within the cortex, specialized regions extract complex scene aspects. Area V1 perceives static form and location. The dorsal stream interprets motion and spatial relationships. The ventral stream identifies color, shape and objects. Surrounding visual association areas integrate inputs for coherent perception and guidance of actions.

Key terminology for discussing the visual apparatus includes common disorders like presbyopia, cataracts, glaucoma and macular degeneration affecting specific structures. Myopia and hyperopia describe refractive errors. Ophthalmic devices include spectacles, contact lenses and intraocular lenses. Analysis of visual function relies on tests assessing acuity, fields, color differentiation and contrast sensitivity. Acuity measures the smallest discernible target, mapped across the visual field, which are quantified by standard eye charts. Automated perimetry examines the field extent. Detailed structure is imaged with techniques like fundoscopy and optical coherence tomography.

In summary, the intricate visual system anatomy mediates light detection, processing of visual features, and perceiving the surrounding world. Each component contributes critical steps enabling functional sight. Mastering the language of vision empowers discussing pathology and effectively applying diagnostic and therapeutic techniques. Fluency with visual system terminology requires repeatedly reinforcing core concepts. Maintaining organized notes, flashcards and diagrams boosts retention. Using terms consistently in clinical discussions cements the connections between vocabulary and practical application.

Seeking opportunities to examine the living human eye builds tangible familiarity with anatomy. Direct ophthalmoscopy practice sharpens understanding of retinal landmarks revealed under magnification. Observing eye surgeries provides experiential learning. Volunteering at vision screening clinics helps associate vocabulary with clinical techniques. Thorough history taking clarifies the patient's visual experience and perceived deficits. Listening for descriptive modifiers that localize pathology to specific structures guides workup. Assessing how daily function is impacted determines appropriate interventions. Checking external structures and inspecting for abnormalities like lid drooping or pupillary irregularities. Dilating eye drops enable comprehensive funduscopic examination, noting retinal lesions suggestive of hypertension, diabetes or degeneration. Visualizing optic nerve head cupping indicates glaucoma. Measuring near point accommodation aids presbyopia evaluation. Assessing visual fields and acuity quantifies defects. Optical coherence tomography, CT and MRI detail posterior segment structures and disorders. Fluorescein angiography highlights retinal vasculature abnormalities. Visual evoked potential testing evaluates optic nerve function. Referral for formal ophthalmology consultation is warranted when examination suggests significant disease requiring specialty expertise.

Integrating vocabulary with clinical evaluation and diagnostic modalities establishes a strong foundation for managing visual complaints. Keeping vision assessment skills sharp through routine practice maintains readiness to recognize subtle abnormalities early when treatment is most effective.

Common Conditions

The intricate structures facilitating sight each contribute unique functions, making the visual system vulnerable to many disorders. Building expertise in recognizing and managing common ophthalmologic diseases optimizes patient care and outcomes. We will explore key categories of visual pathology frequently encountered.

Refractive errors cause blurred vision from light improperly focusing on the retina. Myopia results from excessive refractive power, while hyperopia stems from inadequate refraction. Astigmatism arises from an irregularly curved cornea, while presbyopia results from the aging eye's reduced ability to accommodate. Refractive errors can be corrected withwith spectacles, contact lenses or surgery. Ocular hypertension impairs aqueous humor drainage, increasing intraocular pressure. Chronic elevation damages the optic nerve, causing glaucoma-related visual field loss. Medications and surgery help control pressure to prevent blindness. Detecting characteristic changes in the optic nerve facilitates early diagnosis and intervention. Cataracts cloud the lens, reducing acuity from light scattering. Congenital, traumatic and metabolic disorders underlie some childhood cataracts, while aging causes most adult cases. Surgery to remove and replace the lens restores vision lost to opacity. Preoperative eye measurement optimizes intraocular lens specifications.

Age-related macular degeneration affects the central retina, blurring detail vision from accumulating waste byproducts. The neovascular "wet" form also causes fluid leakage damaging photoreceptors. Anti-VEGF injections may help when caught early. Oxidative stress and genetics likely contribute to pathology. Diabetic retinopathy stems from chronically elevated blood glucose damaging small vessels supplying the retina and disrupting oxygenation. Proliferative disease provokes neovascularization which can hemorrhage or scar. Strict glucose control and intraocular injections help prevent progression to blindness.

In summary, diverse visual disorders arise from inherited anomalies, acquired disease and injury. Each condition impairs distinct aspects of vision in characteristic patterns. Recognizing typical presentations facilitates accurate diagnosis and management. Effective evaluation of these disorders integrates visual acuity testing, external inspection, pupillary response assessment and dilated funduscopic exam. Visual field plotting precisely maps defects; optical coherence tomography visualizes retinal layers and macular anatomy. Fluorescein angiography highlights vascular abnormalities. Tailoring management to the underlying diagnosis is critical. Refractive error correction should precisely match the identified defects. Glaucoma treatment lowers elevated intraocular pressure using medication, laser or surgery while cataract surgery timing balances acuity loss versus surgical risk. Counseling on realistically achievable outcomes ensures appropriate expectations. Preoperative teaching prepares patients for post-surgical care like eyedrop regimens and activity restrictions during healing. Emphasizing compliance with medications and follow-up monitoring helps sustain visual gains.

Supporting patients in adapting to their vision changes helps maximize their remaining vision. Providing tools like magnification, better lighting, and improved contrast makes reading and navigation easier. Teaching patients to use their peripheral vision through eccentric viewing can be very effective. Referring patients to vision rehabilitation offers training in using low vision aids and assistive technologies. Open discussions about the emotional impact and coping techniques ensure holistic care and support.

Integrating clinical findings, diagnostic testing and patient priorities guides the management of these disorders. Keeping current with rapidly evolving therapies ensures that optimal options are being offered. However, established interventions remain foundational while awaiting validation of innovations. Sustained excellence requires lifelong learning and skill refinement.

Diagnostic Procedures

Comprehensively assessing visual function and ocular anatomy facilitates detecting abnormalities early when interventions are most effective. We will explore key techniques for evaluating the visual system, ranging from simple bedside tests to advanced imaging modalities.

The basic visual screening tests include acuity, fields, external exam, pupil reactivity and ophthalmoscopy. Visual acuity measures the smallest discernible target on standardized charts while near vision acuity highlights presbyopia untreated by distance correction. Confrontation visual field testing is used to map defects. External inspection highlights lid position, discharge and conjunctival injection. Pupillary light response detects optic nerve or brainstem dysfunction and direct ophthalmoscopy evaluates retinal vessels and optic nerve. Furthermore, formal visual field testing precisely maps scotomas and deficits. Automated static perimetry uses light stimuli projected across the visual field quantifying detection accuracy while kinetic perimetry employs a moving target to map field borders. Also, selective testing evaluates specific visual pathways and lastlt, serial evaluations monitor changes.

Imaging modalities provide detailed views of ocular structures. Fundus photography documents the appearance of the optic nerve head, while fluorescein angiography highlights retinal vasculature using injected dye. Optical coherence tomography (OCT) offers high-resolution cross-sections of the retina, useful for evaluating the macula. CT scans are used to characterize orbital and bony anatomy, whereas MRI excels at detailing soft tissue without radiation exposure. Additional testing assesses specific functions. Contrast sensitivity evaluation detects early disease affecting daily tasks before acuity loss. The use of color vision testing uncovers congenital or acquired defects. Electroretinography on the another hand, measures retinal response to light. There is also visual evoked potentials which assess optic nerve signals. Finally, ocular motility evaluation examines extraocular movements.

In summary, comprehensive efficient examination relies on selecting appropriate tests based on history and presentation. Results guide targeted advanced testing to determine underlying pathology. Integrating findings provides an accurate diagnosis directing proper management. When seeing patients with visual complaints, methodically moving through a structured examination maximizes detecting subtle findings. Consistently following the same sequence with time, will improve fluency and prevent overlooking important steps.

Starting with acuity assessment highlights defects impacting daily function. Observing while the patient enters the room immediately provides an insight on the navigation ability of the patient. Testing near and distance vision uncovers unique issues. External exam looks for discharge, swelling or asymmetry and pupillary testing notes irregularities. Dilated funduscopic exam visualizes optic nerve head cupping suggestive of glaucoma and retinal abnormalities like hemorrhages. Meticulous documentation facilitates comparison at follow-up. Characterizing scotoma location and quality clarifies possible origins.

Ordering advanced testing guided by clinical concern increases yield. For glaucoma suspicion, visual field plotting and OCT of nerve fiber layer assess damage. Macular degeneration warrants OCT imaging of central retina anatomy. Floaters or photopsias prompt evaluation of retinal holes, tears or detachments. Promptly communicating significant findings to the patient, with counseling on next steps and indication for specialty referral, reduces anxiety and facilitates follow-up compliance. Providing thorough clinical information and examination, documentation to consultants ensures efficient continuity of care.

The Auditory System

Anatomy and Key Terms

Hearing facilitates communication and environmental awareness by translating sound waves into neural signals interpreted by the brain. The structures mediating audition each contribute specialized functions. We will survey core auditory apparatus anatomy and key terminology underlying the sense of hearing.

Sound collection begins at the pinna, which channels sound waves towards the auditory canal terminating at the tympanic membrane. Vibration of the tympanic membrane is transduced to mechanical movement of the ossicular chain, comprised of the malleus, incus and stapes. This mechanical energy is converted into hydraulic motion within the cochlea, a fluid-filled spiral structure selectively tuned to specific frequencies by graded stiffness of the basilar membrane. Sensory hair cells contacting the membrane convert this motion into electrical potentials carried by the auditory nerve. Auditory signals synapse in the cochlear nuclei of the brainstem prior to reaching the inferior colliculus, medial geniculate nucleus of the thalamus, and ultimately the auditory cortex for conscious perception. Parallel pathways mediate sound localization based on timing and intensity differences at the two ears.

Key terminology includes external ear, middle ear and inner ear components. Conduction versus sensorineural hearing loss differentiates outer/middle ear from cochlear/nerve pathology. Audiometry quantifies hearing sensitivity across frequencies to characterize loss profiles. Tympanometry assesses middle ear function.

Common diagnoses like otitis media, otosclerosis and presbycusis disrupt specific sections of the auditory pathway. Noise induced hearing loss initially affects higher frequencies. Temporal bone fractures can damage delicate inner ear structures and Inner ear hair cell loss alters speech discrimination out of proportion to pure tone thresholds.

In summary, the auditory apparatus involves intricate structures to collect, transduce, and interpret sound information essential for communication and spatial awareness. Fluency with anatomical locations and key concepts empowers effective diagnosis and management of hearing disorders. Developing deep familiarity with auditory structures requires repeatedly reinforcing core concepts through active learning strategies. Outlining pathway components from external to inner ear cements flow. Diagrams can also be used to clarify complex three-dimensional anatomy and flashcards associate key terms with definitions.

Seeking opportunities to directly visualize anatomy is invaluable. Observation of otolaryngologic procedures provides orientation to middle and inner ear spaces. Temporal bone dissection labs offer hands-on experience identifying fine structures. Volunteering at audiology clinics connects vocabulary with assessment techniques. Thorough history taking investigates the patient's auditory complaints and functional impacts. Clarifying onset, progression and circumstances eliciting symptoms localizes pathology. Characterizing hearing difficulties in noise versus quiet settings further directs evaluation. Inspection of the external auditory canal and tympanic membrane is performed under microscopy, pneumatic otoscopy assesses tympanic membrane mobility, Weber and Rinne tuning fork testing provides clues to conductive versus sensorineural loss, while whispered voice and finger rub tests screen for gross deficits.

Formal audiometry quantifies hearing sensitivity across speech and pure tone frequencies. Tympanometry evaluates middle ear function, while speech recognition scores help distinguish between conduction and neural loss. Otoacoustic emission testing assesses the integrity of outer hair cells. If concerning findings arise, ordering an MRI or CT scan can further guide management. Integrating anatomy knowledge, vocabulary and clinical techniques establishes a strong foundation for managing hearing disorders and recognizing when specialty referral is indicated. Keeping skills sharp through ongoing learning and assessment maintains readiness to optimize patient outcomes.

Pathologies and Treatments

Hearing loss carries a significant personal and societal impact, this in turn necessitates the awareness of common causes of hearing loss and guides appropriate interventions. We will explore key auditory system disorders frequently encountered as well as management strategies to optimize outcomes.

Conductive hearing impairment arises from external or middle ear pathology obstructing sound transmission. Impacted cerumen is readily treated with irrigation. Otitis media responds to antibiotics and tympanostomy tubes for recurrent cases. Otosclerosis may require stapedectomy surgery to improve stiffening of sound conduction structures. Sensorineural hearing loss stems from inner ear or auditory nerve damage. Noise exposure and aging are common causes. Severity ranges from subtle high-frequency loss to profound deafness. Hearing aids and cochlear implants restore hearing depending on the severity of the deficit. Vestibular schwannoma tumors may cause similar loss. Acute auditory complaints warrant urgent evaluation to identify potentially reversible processes. Sudden sensorineural loss may respond to steroids if treated early but fluctuating loss raises concern for underlying autoimmune inner ear disease. Unilateral conductive loss however, could reflect cholesteatoma and bone erosion requiring prompt intervention.

In summary, maintaining a broad differential and swiftly matching appropriate therapies to confirmed diagnoses is key for preserving auditory function. This requires continuously cultivating expertise across the spectrum of auditory disorders and available management options. A detailed history of hearing difficulties guides efficient evaluation. Asking about tinnitus and balance symptoms provides clues to pathology. Onset, progression, laterality and exacerbating factors all direct workup. Performing a meticulous head and neck exam inspects for structural abnormalities, drainage or masses. Pneumatic otoscopy assesses tympanic membrane mobility. Weber and Rinne testing provides rapid insights into type of impairment.

Formal audiometry thoroughly assesses and characterizes the degree of hearing loss. Tympanometry evaluates middle ear function, while speech recognition scores help distinguish between outer and inner ear pathology. If there are indications such as asymmetric loss, an MRI may be ordered to screen for tumors. Treatment plans are individualized based on examination findings. Impacted cerumen can be removed by irrigation. Hearing aids should be selected and fitted to match the specific deficits revealed on audiometry. Exploring cochlear implant candidacy involves a multidisciplinary team for selection and education.

Patient counseling is quite important throughout evaluation and management. Thorough education about their diagnosis and interventions prevents confusion. Emphasizing realistic expectations and follow-up compliance promotes successful long-term outcomes. Avoiding excessive noise exposure also helps prevent further damage. Innovations like auditory brainstem implants and otoprotective therapies hold promise for the future. However, rigorously validating safety and efficacy through careful study remains imperative before clinical adoption. Meanwhile, applying evidence-based best practices ensures present patients receive optimal available care.

Hearing Tests and Devices

Confirming and characterizing auditory dysfunction relies on a combination of screening exams and specialized diagnostic tests. Amplification devices can significantly improve communication for those experiencing hearing loss. We will explore key techniques for assessing the auditory system and available technologies to enhance sound detection.

The hearing screening assessment starts with observing patient communication difficulties and inspecting the external canal and tympanic membrane. Pneumatic otoscopy assesses eardrum mobility while tuning fork testing provides rapid differentiation of conductive versus sensorineural loss based on loudness comparison between air and bone conduction. Formal audiometry uses calibrated pure tones across the speech frequency range to quantify and profile hearing deficits. Masking contralateral noise during testing prevents false results. Tympanometry characterizes middle ear function through eardrum mobility measurement. Otoacoustic emission testing assesses outer hair cell integrity and speech audiometry clarifies speech discrimination ability.

The results guide the selection and fitting of hearing assistive devices customized to the patient's profile. Basic amplification aids employ microphones, amplifiers and receivers in a compact unit worn behind the ear. More advanced digital programmable models allow customization for different environments. Implantable bone conduction aids the transmission of sound vibration through the skull when ear canal abnormalities preclude air conduction aids. Cochlear implantation is considered in cases of severe to profound sensory hearing loss unresponsive to amplification. The surgically implanted device directly stimulates the auditory nerve through an electrode array inserted into the cochlea. Candidacy relies on multifaceted assessment of residual hearing, imaging, cognitive function and rehabilitation commitment. Thorough counseling ensures appropriate expectations post-activation. Assistive listening systems facilitate communication in challenging environments through specialized microphones and receivers. Infrared systems transmit to receivers worn by the listener. Induction loop systems send magnetic signals captured by hearing aids switched to telecoil mode. Frequency modulation (FM) systems provide more robust performance across distance via radio signals.

In summary, comprehensive assessment provides crucial detail guiding individualized selection of hearing assistive technologies ranging from simple hearing aids to cochlear implant systems. Keeping current on available devices ensures offering patients optimal solutions for overcoming auditory deficits. Hearing loss carries significant negative social, emotional and medical impacts, so expedient and accurate diagnosis is imperative. Using a structured approach beginning with screening builds efficiency.

Taking a thorough history documenting the problems hearing loss causes for the patient provides context. Asking about tinnitus, pain, discharge or dizziness may indicate underlying pathology. Clarifying progression, laterality and exacerbating factors focuses the workup. Performing a meticulous head and neck examination highlights any structural abnormalities or lesions. Pneumatic otoscopy inspects the tympanic membrane for mobility. Weber and Rinne testing differentiates conductive from sensorineural deficits. Basic testing provides a framework for selecting appropriate advanced diagnostics. Formal audiometry thoroughly examines and profiles hearing loss. Tympanometry assesses middle ear function, speech recognition scoring distinguishes conduction from inner ear issues and ordering imaging like MRI is warranted for indications like unilateral loss or neurological symptoms.

Conveying audiogram results and explaining the next steps keeps patients informed and responsive to recommendations. Counseling aids the acceptance of hearing devices and motivates compliance with follow-up care. Clear communication and patient education fosters the best outcomes.

Olfactory and Gustatory Systems

Key Terms and Functions

The chemical senses of smell and taste enrich our perception and enjoyment of food, environments and each other. We will explore the anatomy facilitating these primal yet complex sensory modalities and survey key terminology defining their attributes.

Olfaction relies on specialized olfactory receptor neurons within the upper nasal cavity detecting airborne chemical compounds. Axons of these neurons penetrate the cribriform plate, synapsing in the olfactory bulbs of the brain. This *cranial nerve I mediated sensing* includes orthonasal smelling through the nostrils as well as retronasal olfaction, contributing to flavor perception. Gustation utilizes taste receptor cells clustered within papillae on the tongue surface. Different regions detect primary taste modalities including sweet, sour, salty, bitter and savory umami. Cranial nerves VII, IX and X transmit impulses to the nucleus of the solitary tract in the brainstem for interpretation. Sensory integration of olfactory, gustatory and somatosensory input produces the complex phenomenon of flavor. Top-down cognitive processes like attention and memory further shape individual experiences of smell and taste. Key terminology encompassing these concepts provides a foundation for delving into assessment, diagnosis and management of chemosensory disorders.

In summary, interfacing external chemical sampling with internal sensory transduction and higher cortical processing, the olfactory and gustatory systems participate intimately in nutrition, safety and the overall human experience. Appreciating their anatomy and terminology establishes the groundwork for maintaining these vital sensory functions. Grasping olfactory and gustatory physiology requires focused study across levels from receptors to cortical networks. Diagrams are useful in helping to visualize complex anatomy. Active recall strengthens connections, with mnemonics linking concepts to aid retention. Exploring one's own sensory experiences helps to ground abstract concepts. Seeking direct observations reinforces book learning and observing nasal endoscopy provides orientation to intranasal anatomy. Also, watching formal taste testing offers insight into patient experience and clinical assessment techniques. It's important to attend dissections or prosections of respiratory and upper digestive tract specimens cements concepts.

Thorough history taking investigates onset, progression and characteristics of chemosensory complaints. Clarifying which modalities are affected and stimulus specifics guides diagnosis. Collateral input from family members often proves crucial regarding gradual onset of deficits. Formal testing quantifies the degree of impairment for each modality. Olfaction assessment employs odor identification from standardized kits, gustatory function relies on detection and recognition thresholds for each basic taste and contrasting results reveals sensory versus cognitive deficits. Integrating findings into a focused differential diagnosis and tailored management plan provides optimal care aligned with the patient's priorities and presentation. Maintaining open communication ensures the patient's engagement in shared decision-making.

Related Conditions

Smell and taste disturbances significantly impact quality of life. We will survey key disorders of olfaction and gustation that may be encountered in clinical practice and optimal approaches for diagnosis and management.

Olfactory deficits include anosmia, complete loss, and hyposmia, the reduced ability to smell. Causes generally range from head trauma and viral infection to neurodegenerative illness and normal aging. Thorough assessment establishes etiology guiding treatment and counseling. Smell training therapy also shows promise for some causes. Ageusia reflects total taste loss, while hypoguesia denotes decreased taste sensitivity. Nutritional deficiencies, medications, radiation damage, and nerve injury or disease can all impair gustation. Management of these deficits mostly centers on addressing the underlying causes when possible and adapting to promote safer, more palatable nutrition.

Chemosensory distortions like parosmia or phantosmia, respectively smelling incorrect or phantom odors, warrant evaluation to rule out the possibility of serious neurological conditions. In addition, counseling helps patients adapt to often unsettling symptoms. Some particular medications may offer symptomatic relief in some cases.

Given chemosensory dysfunction frequently overlaps multiple modalities. Maintaining a broad differential diagnosis and conducting a structured evaluation clarifies the precise deficits to target appropriate interventions for the individual patient. Open communication and setting realistic expectations facilitates adjustment. Loss of smell profoundly impacts flavor perception and food enjoyment. It also hinders detecting environmental hazards like gas leaks or smoke, posing serious safety risks. Patients require counseling on compensatory strategies to ensure adequate nutrition, hydration and home safety. Referral to smell training therapy and online support communities may help in coping with these lifestyle changes. Taste distortions or deficits can leave patients struggling to maintain proper nutrition and hydration. Therefore, working to identify preferred tolerable foods and seasonings enables establishing a balanced palatable diet. Ruling out contributory nutritional deficiencies and optimizing any other remediable factors improves outcomes.

For anosmia following upper respiratory infection, smell training provides structured olfactory stimulation that may promote recovery in some patients. There is no strong evidence that supports medication interventions. Counseling focuses on safety precautions and compensation strategies. Ruling out neurological conditions like Parkinson's is imperative. Chemosensory assessment involves psychophysical tests to quantify odor identification, detection thresholds, and taste recognition. Imaging and electrophysiological studies help localize lesions, while bloodwork evaluates nutritional and endocrine status. A multidisciplinary approach optimizes diagnosis and identifies candidates for emerging interventions like neuromodulation.

In summary, smell and taste disorders disrupt nutrition, safety and quality of life. Awareness of common presentations guides a targeted workup and provides counseling tailored to the individual's deficits and priorities, aiming to overcome challenges.

CHAPTER 4

MUSCULOSKELETAL AND INTEGUMENTARY SYSTEMS

Musculoskeletal System Terminology

Bones and Muscles

The musculoskeletal system provides form, stability, locomotion and physical interaction through specialized skeletal, muscular and connective tissues. Fluency with core anatomy and terminology enhances clinical assessment and communication regarding this vital apparatus. We will review key bones, muscles and associated terms to establish a foundational lexicon.

The skeletal system forms from connective tissue into bones classified by shape, feature locations and articulations. Long bones including the femur and humerus comprise the limbs. Short bones like carpals comprise the wrists and ankles. Flat bones such as the sternum and ribs protect thoracic organs. Irregular bones including vertebrae define the spinal column. Specific bone markings serve as muscle attachment sites and form joints. Protuberances include tuberosities, crests and trochanters. Depressions are called fovea or fossae, condyles are rounded articulation surfaces, foramina allow passage of nerves and vessels and canals like the auditory canal encase structures. Muscles contract to produce movement and force While skeletal muscles attach to bones by tendons, controlling locomotion and position. As striated voluntary muscle, contraction is under somatic nervous control. Muscles often work in complementary pairs across joints such as biceps and triceps controlling arm flexion and extension. Muscle names reference location, shape, action or attachments. The quadriceps group extends the knee, comprising four heads. Hamstrings including the biceps femoris flex the knee. Gluteal muscles of the buttocks drive hip and thigh motion, while the trapezius and rhomboids between the scapulae facilitate scapular movements and posture.

Integrating this foundation empowers clinical description of musculoskeletal pain, dysfunction or injury regarding precise anatomical structures. It also enables clear communication with patients about their health. Deepening knowledge of musculoskeletal medicine requires reinforcing core concepts while continually expanding the working lexicon. A crucial step is learning anatomical terminology in both Latin and common forms. Actively labeling diagrams, models and one's own musculoskeletal structures strengthens recollection. Flashcards and repetitive self-testing builds fluency over time and viewing cadaver prosections ties concepts to real anatomy.

Clinical training provides direct hands-on experience. Performing physical exams highlights surface landmarks denoting deeper structures. Assisting in surgery also provides orientation to spaces between muscles and surrounding neurovascular structures needing protection. Experience clarifies textbook knowledge. Obtaining a targeted history focuses the musculoskeletal evaluation. Characterizing the location, quality, onset and aggravating/alleviating factors of reported pain guides assessment. Asking about weakness or limitations in range of motion helps localize affected structures.

Inspection identifies gross deformities, asymmetry or skin changes suggesting underlying pathology. Palpation locates points of tenderness and swelling indicating potential sites of injury. Active and passive range of motion testing assesses the joint and muscle function. There are also special tests like McMurray's maneuver which target specific structures. Integrating findings into a differential diagnosis directs appropriate imaging, specialist referral and treatment to provide optimal patient care while avoiding unnecessary interventions. Clear documentation and patient communication ensures the understanding of anatomy involved.

Joint and Ligament Terms

Joints provide structured articulation between bones, supported by specialized connective tissues to confer stability. Fluency with terms for joint types, features and reinforcing ligament anatomy facilitates clear clinical communication regarding musculoskeletal deficits. We will review key terminology for these integral musculoskeletal components.

Structural joints are classified by mobility. Therefore, synarthroses like sutures of the skull provide little to no movement. However, amphiarthroses such as symphyses allow slight motion and diarthroses including knee and shoulder joints permit free articulation. They are further categorized by a number of articulating bones. Specific diarthroses feature characteristic shapes matching interacting surface anatomy. Hinge joints like the elbow, flex and extend along one axis. Pivot joints on the other hand, such as the atlantoaxial junction rotate around a central point. There are however, condyloid joints including wrist and knuckles which combine flexion, extension and rotation. Ball and socket joints provide maximum mobility through rotation around multiple axes.

The shoulder generally has the greatest range of motion. The hip also supports more weight bearing as a more constrained ball and socket joint. Joint stability arises from static and dynamic elements. Static stabilizers include bony contours along with ligament and joint capsule reinforcement while dynamic stabilization relies on coordinated muscle contractions counteracting forces generated by joint motion. Ligaments consist of dense regular connective tissue that span joints and attach to bone. They prevent or limit certain motions providing passive stability. Collateral ligaments on each side resist side-to-side or varus-valgus forces. Cruciate ligaments cross inside joints to resist rotation. Examples include the ulnar collateral ligament of the elbow and anterior cruciate ligament of the knee. The plantar calcaneonavicular ligament maintains the medial longitudinal foot arch. An Injury typically requires surgical repair after acute tears and gradual wear can lead to degenerative instability.

Integrating the language of joints facilitates localized clinical descriptions of dysfunction related to specific articulations and reinforcing soft tissue restraints. Mastering this foundation allows building advanced expertise to manage complex musculoskeletal pathologies. Joint and ligament terminology can seem daunting at first. But taking time to methodically review each new term, maping it to patient anatomy and using memory techniques to reinforce the concepts enables building competency. Actively labeling joint types and ligament locations on diagrams and models, as well as one's own joints during physical exam practise, aids retention. Creating flashcards for key terms initiates use and repetition reinforcing the lexicon. Observing actual joint structures during rotations, dissections or surgical cases grounds the textbook knowledge in real anatomy. Visualizing the zones of cartilage wear in degenerative arthritis clarifies concepts and experiencing ligament quality differences among specimens of varying ages highlights clinical relevance. Obtaining a thorough history provides clues to involved joints and structures based on described symptoms. Characterizing specific motions that aggravate or alleviate reported pain further localizes pathology. Asking about instability or giving way suggests ligamentous injury.

Performing a comprehensive exam clarifies affected structures. Palpating for swelling and point tenderness indicates potential sites of injury. Assessing range of motion and ligament integrity through varus, valgus and drawer testing detects laxity or deficiencies compared to the uninjured side. Integrating findings into a differential diagnosis considering acuity of injury and chronicity of symptoms guides appropriate imaging, specialist referral and therapy to optimize patient outcomes while minimizing unnecessary interventions.

Common Musculoskeletal Disorders

The musculoskeletal system is vulnerable to a variety of acquired and congenital conditions leading to pain and mobility deficits. We will survey key terminology used to describe common diagnoses involving bones, muscles, joints and supporting connective tissues that may present in clinical practice.

Osteoporosis describes reduced bone mineral density increasing fracture risk, especially in the elderly. Compression fractures of the spine and hip fractures require prompt management to maintain mobility and independence. Vertebral augmentation procedures can provide stabilization. Osteoarthritis reflects progressive degenerative joint changes with articular cartilage loss causing joint space narrowing, osteophyte formation and subchondral sclerosis. It frequently affects the knees, hips and hands causing stiffness, pain and impaired mobility. Total joint arthroplasty can provide significant symptomatic relief in suitable candidates.

Rheumatoid arthritis results from an inflammatory autoimmune process diffusely affecting joints and connective tissues. It manifests with swelling, pain and progressive deformities including ulnar drift of the metacarpophalangeal joints. Early diagnosis and treatment aims to control symptoms and limit disability. Gout describes precipitation of uric acid crystals within joints triggering severe inflammation, classically involving the first metatarsophalangeal joint. Identifying and lowering elevated serum uric acid levels provides effective management of this excruciating arthritic condition. Muscular dystrophies denote inherited disorders featuring progressive wasting and weakness of skeletal muscles. Duchenne muscular dystrophy presents itself in childhood with a characteristic waddling gait and pseudo-hypertrophy of the calves. Supportive care aims to maintain mobility and respiratory function for as long as possible.

Integrating this terminology allows communicating clearly regarding common musculoskeletal diagnoses, needed workup and expectations regarding disease course and management options. Building vocabulary also expands the capacity to provide optimal care aligned with patient priorities. Grasping musculoskeletal terminology requires dedicated study and repetition to reinforce concepts. Actively labeling diagrams of affected anatomy aids retention, creating flashcards facilitates self-testing anywhere and viewing images depicting characteristic radiographic findings cements recognition. It's important to note that clinical exposure proves invaluable. Performing musculoskeletal exams highlights surface landmarks and variations in range of motion. Observing procedures like joint injections provides orientation to joint anatomy and participating in rehabilitation sessions clarifies effective strengthening approaches.

Obtaining a thorough history investigating pain characteristics, trauma, family history and associated symptoms guides diagnosis. Plain films quantify joint space and bone integrity. The use of lab testing confirms inflammatory markers and conditions like gout, while genetic testing identifies inherited conditions. Palpation localizes tenderness and swelling, suggesting involved joints or muscles. Assessment of posture, gait and mobility highlights limitations and asymmetry. Strength and range of motion clarifies functional deficits to quantify. Provocative maneuvers can localize sources of impingement.

Synthesizing findings while referencing current guidelines facilitates developing individualized management integrating pharmacological, interventional, physical therapy and surgical options as indicated to provide optimal care while setting realistic expectations.

Integumentary System Terminology

Skin, Hair, and Nails

The integumentary system comprises the skin, hair, nails and associated structures. This protective barrier safeguards inner tissues while facilitating sensation and temperature regulation. We will survey key terminology describing the anatomy and physiology of these critical surface coverings.

The skin is a complex organ with multiple layers. The epidermis consists of stratified squamous epithelium including keratinized surface cells limiting water loss. The thicker dermis underneath contains fibrous and elastic tissues supplying strength and flexibility along with sensory nerves and vasculature. The skin serves diverse functions from sensation to temperature regulation facilitated by associated structures. Appendages of the skin include hair follicles, nails, sebaceous glands and sweat glands. Eccrine sweat glands opening through pores help dissipate heat stimulated by autonomic innervation. Sebaceous glands secrete oily sebum providing waterproofing and sun protection. Vellus hairs cover the body while terminal hairs grow more thickly in regions like the scalp. Hair shafts project above the surface while roots anchored in follicles receive sensory nerve fibers. Fingernails and toenails are composed of keratin produced by the nail matrix extending the nail plate over the nail bed. Cuticles provide protective barriers where the nail plate meets the surrounding skin. It's important to note that the flow of nutrients through the nail bed will impact growth and health.

Mastering terminology for the integumentary system establishes a foundation for clinical assessment and communication regarding the wide range of skin disorders and injuries that may be present in practice. Fluency with associated vocabulary supports providing optimal dermatologic care. Building expertise requires methodical vocabulary expansion through studying diagrams, undertaking self-testing and actively labeling one's own integumentary anatomy during skin exams. Review sessions with flash cards facilitate memorization of new terms and seeing dermatologic pathology samples reinforces connections between visual findings and descriptive terminology.

Clinical rotations provide invaluable direct experience. Assisting with wound care clarifies terms describing ulcers, drainage and healing. Performing full skin exams highlights surface morphology variations and normal patterns. Participating in procedures like cyst excisionscan aid in cementing the understanding of subsurface anatomy. A targeted history noting characteristics, distribution, exacerbating and alleviating factors guides the assessment of skin complaints. A thorough head to toe inspection will clarify primary, secondary and localized findings potentially indicative of systemic conditions. Palpating for induration, tenderness and fluctuance detects abnormalities. Skin scrapings, punch biopsies and culture inform microscopic findings and sensitivities directing treatment. Bloodwork assesses for contributors like nutritional deficiencies, infective causes and autoimmune conditions warranting immunomodulatory therapy. Integrating findings with consideration of patient risk factors and priorities, shapes appropriate referral, non-invasive and interventional treatment planning to provide optimal individualized dermatologic care.

Common Dermatological Terms

The integumentary system is vulnerable to numerous acquired and congenital conditions that may present with skin, nail or hair manifestations. We will survey key terminology used to describe common dermatologic diagnoses likely to be encountered in clinical practice.

Atopic dermatitis refers to a chronic, pruritic inflammatory skin condition featuring erythema, lichenification and excoriations which often follows a flexural distribution. It typically starts in childhood with fluctuating severity and is frequently associated with other atopic diseases like asthma. Topical anti-inflammatory treatments form the mainstay of management. Psoriasis denotes an immune-mediated disorder causing thick, scaly plaques with a predilection for the extensor surface of extremities, scalp and lumbosacral regions. The chronic relapsing course often requires rotating systemic therapies to achieve adequate control and improve quality of life given significant psychosocial impact. Acne vulgaris describes the exceedingly common condition of open and closed comedones, inflammatory papules and pustules and nodular cysts resulting from excess sebum, follicular hyperkeratinization and proliferation of Propionibacterium acnes. Topical and oral treatments target pathogenesis. The possiblity of acarring warrants prevention. Urticaria refers to pruritic, raised edematous wheals ranging in size from a few millimeters to several inches across. It often manifests acutely following allergic triggers but can present as chronic idiopathic urticaria. Avoidance measures and antihistamines provide symptomatic relief. Angioedema denotes similar deep dermal edema. Melanoma represents potentially lethal cutaneous malignancy derived from melanocytes which most often appears as asymmetric, irregularly pigmented lesions with color variegation. Early detection and excision is imperative to reduce morbidity and mortality from this aggressive cancer with its propensity for metastasis.

Incorporating this vocabulary enables communicating clearly regarding common integumentary pathologies to provide optimal patient education, counseling and care aligned with treatment guidelines and individual circumstances. Grasping dermatologic terminology requires concerted study and repetition. Actively labeling diagrams strengthens visual recognition of characteristic findings, flashcards aid in mastering definitions and viewing clinical photographs grounds concepts in real patient presentations. Rotations offer direct opportunities to refine the working lexicon. Hearing attendings describe findings cements new phrases. Participating in procedures like skin biopsies links terminology to histopathology. Clinic experience connects textbook knowledge to actual practice.

Obtaining a focused history noting lesion progression, associated symptoms and pertinent risk factors guides diagnosis. A full body scan identifies all primary and secondary skin findings. Palpation assesses for induration, tenderness and fluctuance and dermoscopy aids in evaluating pigmented lesions. Skin scrapings, punch biopsies and viral culture help elucidate microscopic and molecular characteristics of rashes guiding therapy. Bloodwork evaluates for underlying causes like infection, autoimmune conditions and nutritional deficiency.

Integrating clinical data and patient priorities with current guidelines enables developing individualized management plans to optimize outcomes. Checking patient comprehension ensures adherence and follow up.

Diagnostic and Treatment Procedures

The integumentary system lends itself to a broad array of diagnostic and therapeutic interventions facilitating targeted management of skin disorders. We will review key terminology pertaining to common dermatologic procedures clinicians may perform or refer patients to.

Diagnostic modalities aid lesion assessment. Dermoscopy involves examining skin lesions under magnification with fluid and polarized light to visualize morphological characteristics in greater detail to enhance diagnostic accuracy. It can help differentiate benign nevi from melanoma. Skin biopsy refers to sampling a portion of skin lesion for microscopic histopathologic examination to confirm the diagnosis and guide definitive treatment. Punch, shave and excisional biopsies remove varying amounts of tissue based on the indication and location. Curettage involves sharp debridement of growths down to the dermal layer.

Culture, staining and immunofluorescence help identify infectious causes and immunobullous disorders. Skin scrapings and hair examinations detect parasites. While provocative allergy testing assesses for contact sensitivities, Imaging like ultrasound evaluates the extent of deeper processes. Topical medications comprise first-line treatments for most dermatoses. Emollients hydrate and protect the skin barrier, corticosteroids reduce inflammation, calcineurin inhibitors modulate immunity and keratolytics exfoliate to diminish plaques. Also, antifungals, antibiotics and antivirals target underlying infections. Intralesional injections deliver medication directly into lesions. Triamcinolone ameliorates inflammation while 5-fluorouracil stimulates necrosis of growths. Hyaluronidase enhances diffusion in collagenosis and electroporation facilitates topical uptake. Botulinum toxin also reduces excessive sweating.

Surgical approaches are often indicated for removals, reconstructions and aesthetic enhancement. Excision extirpates benign and malignant lesions, cryosurgery freezes tissue causing necrosis and curettage involves sharp debridement. Laser therapy permits precise tissue ablation while dermabrasion refines appearance.

Integrating this foundation empowers accurate documentation and effective patient communication regarding dermatologic procedures under consideration for their care. Mastering the terminology therefore enables clear discussions of risks, benefits, expectations and follow up needs associated with recommended interventions. Building expertise in discussing procedures requires concerted effort to expand one's lexicon. Studying images and illustrations clarifies nuances between techniques. Observing clinics and surgeries often offer exposure to actual methods. Role-playing conversations facilitates natural integration into practice dialogue. Clinical training opportunities prove invaluable. Assisting with biopsies cements foundational skills in anesthesia and closure methods. Performing cryotherapy strengthens procedural competency and following treatment response helps correlate interventions with outcomes to better inform care planning.

A targeted history identifies lesions and impacts needing intervention. Inspection characterizes morphology and distribution of findings. Palpation detects induration, tenderness or fluctuance. Diagnostic testing shapes definitive procedural plans when conservative treatments prove insufficient. Thoughtfully weighing risks, benefits, costs and expected outcomes for the individual patient in context of current guidelines enables devising appropriate treatment plans. Ensuring patient understanding regarding realistic expectations, proper aftercare, and follow-up needs optimizes procedural success and improves adherence to integrate recommendations into long-term management.

CHAPTER 5

REPRODUCTIVE AND ENDOCRINE SYSTEMS

Reproductive System

Male and Female Systems

Reproduction depends on intricate physiologic coordination between specialized male and female reproductive structures to perpetuate the species. We will survey key terminology describing the anatomy and function of these complementary systems.

The male reproductive system comprises the testes, epididymis, vas deferens, seminal vesicles and penis. The penis consists of the root, shaft, and glans. The foreskin or prepuce covers the glans. The testes produce sperm and testosterone supported by cells in the seminiferous tubules and interstitial tissue. An erection occurs when the paired corpora cavernosa fills with blood and the epididymis stores and transports sperm toward the vas deferens. Accessory sex glands include the seminal vesicles contributing fructose for sperm metabolism and prostate secreting alkaline fluid. The corpus spongiosum surrounds the spongy urethra which transports urine and semen. During ejaculation, the semen is propelled through the urethra.

The major female reproductive organs are the ovaries, uterine tubes, uterus and vagina. The ovaries produce ova supported by follicular cells. The follicular phase culminating in ovulation follows the menstrual proliferative phase stimulated by FSH and estrogen. The fallopian tubes provide conduits for ova toward the uterus aided by cilia and peristalsis. The uterus features an inner endometrium lining that thickens during the secretory phase under progesterone influence to support potential implantation. The vagina receives the penis during intercourse and serves as the birth canal. External genitalia include the mons pubis, clitoris, urethral meatus and labia. Breast anatomy includes the nipple, areola, lactiferous ducts and glandular tissue.

Integrating foundational reproductive terminology establishes a basis for clear clinical communication regarding patient symptoms, examination findings and potential pathologies of these delicate systems.

Comprehending reproductive language relies on reinforcing self-study. Labeling diagrams aids visual identification, making flashcards links terms to definitions, answering practice questions cements details and direct clinical exposure proves invaluable. Also, observing reproductive exams and procedures grants orientation to anatomy. Following complex cases reinforces nuances. Clinical rotations build practical connections between terminology and real patient assessments.

A thorough history evaluating pubertal onset, sexual activity, symptoms like discharge or pain, and reproductive goals guides evaluation. Physical exam assesses external genitalia and internal structures like the cervix. Targeted lab testing elucidates function. Semen analysis evaluates sperm, hormone levels identify deficiencies, imaging details structural abnormalities, endoscopy permits direct visualization and biopsies characterize lesions. Synthesizing findings considering the patient's circumstances and preferences enables developing individualized management plans encompassing fertility assistance, hormonal treatments, counseling or surgical intervention as appropriate. Ongoing care emphasizes education regarding safe sexual practices, regular screening, and prompt reporting of concerning symptoms to promote reproductive health.

Key Reproductive Health Terms

Optimizing reproductive health over the lifespan requires a working knowledge of terminology pertaining to associated physiologic processes, common disorders and recommended preventive care. We will survey key terms frequently encountered when addressing reproductive wellbeing.

Puberty denotes the period of physical maturation resulting from hormonal changes in which adolescents develop secondary sex characteristics and attain fertility. Supporting adolescents through pubertal changes is crucial for social-emotional wellbeing. Menstruation refers to the cyclical shedding of the uterine lining that occurs in women typically beginning in early puberty until menopause. Menopause represents the cessation of menses marking the end of fertility. Perimenopause is the transition period leading up to menopause when cycles become irregular. Symptoms like hot flashes and vaginal atrophy often prompt treatment during this time. Regular menstrual cycles range from 21-35 days averaging 28 days. Abnormal uterine bleeding warrants evaluation.

Contraception describes methods for preventing pregnancy. Options include barrier methods like condoms, hormonal methods like oral contraceptives, intrauterine devices, sterilization procedures and natural family planning techniques. The most effective choices are long-acting reversible contraceptives. Prenatal care encompasses medical supervision during pregnancy to monitor fetal growth and maternal health. It includes regular obstetric visits, diagnostic screening and counseling regarding nutrition, exercise and avoiding teratogens. Good prenatal care improves outcomes.

Infertility refers to the inability to achieve pregnancy after a year of regular unprotected intercourse. It affects 10-15% of couples with contributing male and female factors. Treatment modalities include medical management, intrauterine insemination and assisted reproductive technologies like in vitro fertilization.

Sexually transmitted infections (STIs) represent common bacterial, viral and parasitic infections spread through sexual contact affecting reproductive health. Early detection and treatment prevents complications. Using condoms during sexual intercouse provides protection against STIs. Well-woman care refers to recommended regular preventive health visits including cancer screening, STI testing, contraceptive counseling, and discussions regarding reproductive health goals and concerns. Scheduling annual well-woman exams promotes longevity and quality of life. Prescribing appropriate health maintenance requires fluency in reproductive terminology. Discussing concerns, counseling patients and clarifying treatment risks and benefits relies on a nuanced working lexicon covering anatomy, physiology and associated disorders. Ongoing learning from quality resources and colleagues reinforces competency. Clinical exposure cements comprehension, completing the transition from textbook definitions to practical mastery.

Fertility and Reproductive Technologies

For patients challenged with infertility, advanced technologies offer hope for achieving parenthood. We will explore key terminology and concepts related to assisted reproduction.

Infertility refers to the inability to achieve pregnancy after one year of regular intercourse without contraception or six months for women over 35. About 10-15% of couples are affected due to female factors like anovulation, tubal problems or endometriosis and male factors like low sperm count or dysfunction. Initial testing evaluates ovulation, uterine and tubal anatomy and patency and semen quality. Treatment aims to address identified abnormalities, and may begin with ovulation induction medications like clomiphene citrate. Intrauterine insemination (IUI) involves injecting processed, concentrated sperm directly into the uterus around ovulation. Success rates per cycle are modest but costs are lower than in vitro options.

In vitro fertilization (IVF) encompasses retrieval of multiple oocytes after ovarian stimulation followed by fertilization with sperm outside the body, then transferring the resulting embryo(s) into the uterus. Younger women with good quality embryos have the best outcomes. Intracytoplasmic sperm injection (ICSI) represents a specialized IVF technique that involves direct injection of a single sperm into each oocyte using micromanipulation when semen parameters are poor. Fertilization and pregnancy rates improve.

Surrogacy refers to one woman (the surrogate) carrying and giving birth to a baby for another individual or couple (the intended parent(s)) when physiological limitations would prevent safe pregnancy. Traditional vs gestational delineates whether or not the surrogate's own egg is used. Legal contracts outline responsibilities and rights. Donor eggs, sperm or embryos may enable parenthood when one or both partners' gametes are not viable options. Donors usually undergo medical and genetic screening. The degree of future involvement and disclosure to offspring varies based on preferences.

Cryopreservation facilitates the storage of extra embryos following IVF or donor eggs/sperm for future cycles. Slow freezing or newer vitrification both allow successful thawing for transfer later. Preimplantation genetic testing involves screening embryos for chromosomal abnormalities or inherited disorders prior to transferring only unaffected ones, improving IVF success rates. While costs are considerable and success not guaranteed, these technologies enable many with infertility to fulfill their dreams of growing their families when natural conception is not possible. Careful patient selection and counseling ensures realistic expectations. Ongoing innovation aims to continuously improve outcomes while minimizing risks. For suitable candidates, reproductive medicine can be tremendously empowering, conveying hope and restoring reproductive autonomy.

Endocrine System

Glands and Hormones

The endocrine system regulates nearly all physiologic processes in the body through the coordinated release of specialized hormones from diffuse glandular tissue and discrete glands. We will overview key glands and associated hormones critical for homeostasis.

The hypothalamus and pituitary gland coordinate the endocrine system. The hypothalamus integrates inputs and releases hormones that stimulate or inhibit pituitary release of hormones like growth hormone, thyroid stimulating hormone, adrenocorticotropic hormone and gonadotropins for the reproductive axis. The pineal gland secretes melatonin which regulates circadian rhythms and sleep cycles. Insufficient melatonin causes disruption that contributes to medical and psychiatric disease. Supplementation can help recalibrate rhythms in some cases. The thyroid gland produces thyroid hormone (TH), principally thyroxine (T4) and triiodothyronine (T3), that regulates metabolism, growth, and maturation. Low TH causes hypothyroidism while excess causes hyperthyroidism. Monitoring TSH screens for dysfunction.

The parathyroids release parathyroid hormone (PTH) which elevates calcium levels by promoting osteoclast bone resorption and renal calcium reabsorption. Hypoparathyroidism causes hypocalcemia while hyperparathyroidism results in hypercalcemia with associated complications. The adrenal glands have a cortex that produces corticosteroid hormones like glucocorticoids such as cortisol and mineralocorticoids like aldosterone, and a medulla that secretes catecholamines like epinephrine and norepinephrine. These hormones regulate metabolism, inflammation, blood pressure and stress adaptation.

The pancreas contains alpha and beta islet cells that secrete glucagon and insulin respectively. These hormones work in balance to maintain normal glucose levels and fuel delivery. Dysregulation leads to diabetes mellitus.

Gonads refer to the ovaries and testes which produce sex hormones including estrogens, progestins and androgens essential for sexual development and function. Imbalances underlie many reproductive system disorders.

Integrating the fundamentals of endocrine glands and hormones establishes a framework for conceptualizing the far-reaching impacts these chemical messengers exert throughout the body. Recognizing patterns of dysfunction and compensatory mechanisms provides the basis for rational diagnostic evaluation and targeted treatment.

Common Endocrine Disorders

The endocrine system is vulnerable to various disorders resulting from hormonal imbalances. We will survey key terminology pertaining to frequently encountered endocrine diseases and associated clinical presentations.

Diabetes mellitus refers to relative or absolute deficiencies in insulin, resulting in hyperglycemia. Type 1 diabetes is due to autoimmune destruction of beta cells while type 2 results from target tissue insulin resistance and inadequate compensatory insulin secretion. Both cause vascular complications if poorly controlled. Hypothyroidism denotes an underactive thyroid gland leading to reduced metabolic rate, fatigue, cold intolerance, constipation and fluid retention. Hashimoto's thyroiditis often underlies this condition. Replacement thyroid hormone reverses symptoms and prevents sequelae. Hyperthyroidism on the other hand, stems from thyroid overactivity, most commonly from Graves' disease, causing weight loss, tachycardia, tremors and agitation. Antithyroid drugs, radioactive iodine and surgery aim to reduce thyroid function in this setting.

Adrenal insufficiency, known as Addison's disease, arises when the adrenal glands inadequately produce glucocorticoids and mineralocorticoids, resulting in hypotension, fatigue, anorexia and electrolyte abnormalities. Cortisol replacement prevents crises. Cushing's syndrome refers to the effects of prolonged, inappropriately high exposure to cortisol, which can arise from pituitary or adrenal tumors. Features include central obesity, thinning skin, poor wound healing and emotional changes. Treatment aims to reduce cortisol levels.

Hyperparathyroidism manifests when excess PTH secretion by a benign tumor leads to hypercalcemia with resultant kidney stones, bone pain and fractures. Definitive treatment involves surgical removal of the adenoma. Endocrine cancers pose additional challenges. Thyroid cancer risk stratification guides decisions between surgical and medical management. Testicular cancer often requires chemotherapy. Adrenal tumors must be differentiated as benign or malignant based on biopsy findings. Pancreatic cancer has a poor prognosis.

Polycystic ovarian syndrome (PCOS) presents with menstrual irregularity, infertility, obesity and hyperandrogenism in reproductive aged women. Lifestyle modifications combined with medications like metformin and oral contraceptives provide symptom relief and reduce complications.

Integrating foundational pathology equips clinicians to recognize characteristic presentations, order appropriate diagnostic studies, synthesize findings and initiate suitable therapies targeting the root endocrine imbalance to restore normal physiology. Knowledge empowers skillful management of complex endocrine disease.

Diagnostic and Management Approaches

Establishing an accurate endocrine diagnosis and implementing effective management requires methodical synthesis of clinical presentation, physical findings, targeted diagnostic studies and monitoring of treatment responses. We will review strategic approaches to evaluation and management of endocrine disorders.

A thorough history documenting symptoms, comorbidities, medications and family history provides initial clues pointing toward a particular endocrine pathology. Key details include onset and progression, aggravating and relieving factors and impacts on quality of life. The clinical picture guides judicious selection of laboratory and imaging tests. Baseline screening includes a metabolic panel assessing glucose, electrolytes, kidney and liver function. Thyroid studies check TSH and free T4 levels. Suspected abnormalities merit additional testing guided by the differential diagnosis. Provocative stimulation or suppression protocols confirm dysfunction.

Dynamic testing assessments target gland response to specified stimuli. For example, ACTH stimulation tests adrenal cortisol reserve and TRH stimulation evaluates pituitary TSH release. Glucose tolerance testing characterizes diabetes severity by quantifying insulin secretion patterns. Imaging modalities such as ultrasound, CT and MRI visualize structural glandular changes and identify lesions. Nuclear medicine studies like radionuclide scanning provide functional detail. Biopsies are occasionally needed for histopathologic diagnosis, particularly regarding malignancies.

Treatment aims to remedy hormone deficits or excess. Replacement therapy provides missing hormones such as thyroxine, insulin and testosterone. Medications block synthesis or receptor activation to reduce high levels of hormones. Surgery, radiation or chemotherapy target cancers. Ongoing management emphasizes lifestyle optimization, monitoring for complications, adjusting medication dosing in response to changing requirements and ensuring adherence. Patients require education about their condition. Meticulous follow up care improves outcomes.

Endocrinology epitomizes precision medicine, integrating demographics, symptoms, exam findings and investigations to pinpoint specific dysfunction, then guiding therapy selection based on the root pathology and its nuances in each unique individual. Clinical acumen combines with compassion to address both disease and patient in a holistic manner. The rewards of correctly unraveling puzzling presentations and restoring wellbeing are immense.

CHAPTER 6

INFECTIONS, ONCOLOGY, AND PHARMACOLOGICAL TERMS

Infectious Diseases

Key Terms and Pathogen Types

Infectious diseases remain a major cause of morbidity and mortality worldwide. Mastering associated terminology provides a strong foundation for understanding these diverse illnesses. We will overview key concepts and pathogen classifications central to the study of infections and host defenses.

Infectious diseases result from pathogenic microorganisms such as viruses, bacteria, fungi and parasites. Transmission occurs through direct or indirect contact, airborne inhalation, fecal-oral, bloodborne, sexual contact or vector-borne routes. Virulence refers to a pathogen's ability to establish infection and cause damage. Many factors contribute including adhesins, toxins, antigenic variability and invasive enzymes. Host immunity and genetics also influence susceptibility. Colonization means pathogens multiply without tissue invasion or damage. Infection denotes organisms invading and proliferating in host cells, eliciting immune responses. Disease results when cellular injury causes clinical symptoms. Carriers harbor organisms without symptoms.

Viruses possess genetic material surrounded by a protein coat. As obligate intracellular parasites, they require host cells for replication. RNA viruses include influenza, measles and HIV. DNA viruses include herpesviruses, hepatitis B and adenoviruses. Bacteria are prokaryotic cells with peptidoglycan cell walls, circular DNA and no membrane-bound organelles. Many produce toxins and enzymes enhancing virulence. Examples include Streptococcus, Clostridium and Mycobacterium. Rickettsia are bacteria that live in arthropods, transmitted by bites or feces. These include Rocky Mountain spotted fever and typhus. Chlamydia and mycoplasma lack cell walls with cholesterol membranes and limited metabolism.

Spirochetes feature axial filaments enabling corkscrew motility. Treponema causes syphilis, borrelia burgdorferi transmits Lyme disease and leptospira interrogans causes leptospirosis. Mycobacteria have thick waxy cell walls containing mycolic acids. Mycobacterium tuberculosis causes tuberculosis and atypical mycobacteria are environmental organisms causing opportunistic disease. Fungi are eukaryotes that obtain nutrients through absorption. Superficial fungi include dermatophytes affecting skin, hair and nails. Systemic mycoses like histoplasmosis and coccidioidomycosis infect deeper tissues.

Parasites live on or within hosts, consuming nutrients and causing illness. Intestinal parasites are paraites that can be transmitted via fecal-oral contact. Protozoa include Giardia intestinalis and Plasmodium falciparum causing malaria. Helminths are multicellular worms. Prions lack nucleic acids, composed entirely of misfolded prion proteins leading to neurodegenerative illnesses like Creutzfeldt-Jakob disease. Transmission occurs from exposure to contaminated tissue.

Comprehending characteristics of diverse pathogens provides context for understanding the nature of resulting infectious diseases, transmission risks, clinical manifestations and therapeutic approaches. This foundation enables building epidemiologic knowledge, diagnostic acumen and management expertise.

Antibiotics and Treatments

Effectively managing infectious diseases relies on selecting optimal antimicrobial therapy tailored to the causative pathogen and sensitivities, along with addressing complications and host immune factors. We will overview key classes of antibiotics and highlight evolving treatments for major infections.

Penicillins like amoxicillin, interfere with bacterial cell wall synthesis and are first-line drugs for streptococcal pharyngitis, pneumococcal pneumonia and endocarditis. Cephalosporins have expanded gram-negative coverage and β-lactamase inhibitors combat resistance. Macrolides like azithromycin, inhibit protein synthesis to treat atypical respiratory pathogens. Ketolides are similar but have activity against some macrolide-resistant organisms. Oxazolidinones like linezolid, are protein synthesis inhibitors reserved for drug-resistant gram-positive infections.

Fluoroquinolones like ciprofloxacin block DNA replication and are broad-spectrum but reserved when safer options suffice, given side effects. Aminoglycosides like gentamicin have aerobic gram-negative activity but require monitoring for nephrotoxicity and ototoxicity. Glycopeptides like vancomycin target gram-positive cell walls and are used for methicillin-resistant Staphylococcus aureus (MRSA). Newer lipoglycopeptides like dalbavancin offer convenient once-weekly dosing options. Antifungals treat invasive mycoses, azoles like fluconazole inhibit ergosterol synthesis in fungal cell membranes and target yeasts and echinocandins like caspofungin disrupt cell wall glucan synthesis and combat resistant species.

Antiretrovirals are used to suppress HIV replication. Combination agents target viral entry, reverse transcription, integration, and protease enzymes. Highly active antiretroviral therapy (HAART) can dramatically improve prognosis and survival. Hepatitis C antivirals like sofosbuvir, ledipasvir and velpatasvir target key viral proteins resulting in sustained virologic response. Direct acting agents replaced interferon-based regimens with improved efficacy and tolerability.

Influenza treatment relies on neuraminidase inhibitors like oseltamivir when started early, along with emerging antivirals. Supportive care addresses complications like pneumonia. Universal vaccination remains key for prevention.

Understanding foundational antibiotic classes and evolving therapies for major infectious diseases facilitates selection of guideline-concordant, effective treatment tailored to the clinical scenario, improving patient outcomes and combating resistance.

Oncological Terminology

Types of Cancer

Cancer comprises a heterogeneous group of diseases characterized by uncontrolled cellular proliferation. Understanding key terminology provides context for classifying cancers based on cell type, location, growth patterns and spread. This foundation enables understanding risk factors, clinical features, prognostic implications and treatment approaches for different malignancies.

Carcinogenesis entails gradual accumulation of genetic mutations conferring selective growth advantage, evasion of cell cycle regulation and apoptosis, immortality, angiogenesis, invasion and metastasis. Oncogenes activate proliferation while tumor suppressor genes normally inhibit it. Benign tumors are self-limited expansile masses that do not invade surrounding tissues or metastasize, often encapsulated. Malignant cancers exhibit tissue invasion and potential for metastatic spread via lymphatics and blood vessels to distant sites. Staging describes extent of disease based on tumor size, involvement of adjacent structures and presence of metastases.

Carcinoma arises from epithelial tissue and accounts for 80-90% of cancers. Adenocarcinomas develop from glandular epithelium as in cancers of the pancreas, colon and lung. Squamous cell carcinoma affects squamous epithelium such as skin and cervix while transitional cell carcinomas involve the urinary bladder lining. Sarcomas develop from connective tissue or mesenchymal cells. Types include osteosarcoma of bone, leiomyosarcoma of smooth muscle, liposarcoma of fat tissue, and rhabdomyosarcoma of skeletal muscle.

Hematologic cancers originate from blood cell precursors in bone marrow or mature blood cells. Leukemias manifest as a proliferative buildup of abnormal white blood cells. Lymphomas affect lymph nodes and lymphatic channels. Multiple myeloma involves malignant plasma cells accumulating in the bone marrow.

Central nervous system cancers arise from glial cells or coverings like meninges. Gliomas and glioblastomas are aggressive primary brain tumors. Other examples may include medulloblastoma, meningioma, schwannoma and neuroblastoma.

Identifying key features of major cancer categories provides a framework for approaching diagnosis, staging, prognostication, and management. Ongoing research aims to elucidate biological distinctions guiding targeted therapies towards personalized precision medicine.

Terms for Diagnosis and Treatment

Mastering oncology vocabulary is essential for clear communication regarding cancer diagnosis, staging, treatment and prognosis. We will define key terminology pertaining to investigative modalities, surgical interventions, medication classes and outcomes.

Pathology analysis of biopsies and surgical resection specimens confirms malignancy and cancer type based on microscopic appearance, immunophenotyping and genetic markers. Staging relies on imaging like CT, PET and MRI to delineate local vs distant spread guiding treatment. Surgical oncology focuses on removing solid tumors with clear margins. For instance, a lumpectomy excises breast cancer, while a colectomy resects colon cancer. Cytoreductive debulking is performed to optimize the chemotherapy response in ovarian cancer. Additionally, lymph node dissections are done to sample regional drainage patterns. Medical oncology centers on systemic chemotherapy, targeted agents, immunotherapy and hormonal therapy. Cytotoxic chemo targets rapidly dividing cells but affects the healthy ones too. Also, Targeted biologics inhibit specific molecular pathways dysregulated in particular cancers. Hormonal manipulation treats cancers expressing hormone receptors like breast and prostate cancer using anti-estrogens and androgen deprivation while immunotherapy activates the patient's own immune system against the cancer cells. There is also radiation oncology which uses high energy radiation to kill tumor cells and shrink lesions. Linear accelerator external beam radiation focuses beams on the cancer and brachytherapy delivers radioactive seeds inside or next to tumors. Palliative interventions provide pain relief and support when a cure is not possible. Analgesics treat cancer pain, while bisphosphonates strengthen bones weakened by metastases. Antiemetics help mitigate nausea from chemotherapy, and emotional support aids in coping with the illness.

Tumor response criteria gauge treatment efficacy. Complete response signifies that the cancer has disappeared and partial response indicates tumor shrinkage of 30% or more. Stable disease means there has been no significant change while progressive disease denotes continued growth. Remission means apparent elimination of the detectable malignancy. NED (no evidence of disease) indicates complete response sustained over time without relapse. Recurrence after remission is relapse while return after complete response is recurrence.

Surveillance and survivorship care involve monitoring for recurrence through exams, imaging and tumor markers along with managing any long term effects. Support groups and rehabilitation can help with adjustment.

Assimilating cancer terminology transforms complex information into clear communication to guide all stakeholders through the diagnosis and treatment journey for the best outcomes.

Pharmacology

Drug Classifications

Pharmacology encompasses the study of medications, their mechanisms of action, effects and interactions within the body. Understanding drug classifications provides a framework for approaching clinical therapeutics across medical specialties. We will overview major drug categories and representative agents.

Analgesics treat pain arising from inflammation, tissue injury or nerve damage. Non-steroidal anti-inflammatory drugs (NSAIDs) like ibuprofen inhibit cyclooxygenase enzymes reducing prostaglandin production. Opioids like morphine howeer, bind opioid receptors in the brain and spinal cord to block pain signaling. Antimicrobials combat infections. Antibacterials like penicillins, fluoroquinolones and sulfonamides disrupt bacterial cell wall, protein or folate synthesis. Antivirals like acyclovir and oseltamivir inhibit viral DNA polymerase or neuraminidase enzymes and antifungals like fluconazole inhibit fungal cell membrane ergosterol synthesis.

Anticoagulants reduce clotting which can cause thromboembolic events like myocardial infarction and stroke. Warfarin antagonizes vitamin K dependent clotting factors while heparin enhances antithrombin to inhibit thrombin and factor Xa. Direct oral anticoagulants like apixaban directly inhibit thrombin or factor Xa. Proton pump inhibitors like omeprazole suppress gastric acid secretion by blocking H+/K+ ATPase in parietal cells to treat reflux and ulcers. H2 receptor antagonists like ranitidine inhibit histamine stimulated acid production. Antacids like calcium carbonate neutralize stomach acid.

Inhalers are used to treat respiratory diseases. Bronchodilators like albuterol relax airway smooth muscle to relieve bronchospasm in asthma and COPD. Corticosteroids reduce airway inflammation. Mucolytics like acetylcysteine are used to break up mucus secretions.

Hormonal agents modulate endocrine system activity. Estrogens, progestins, and androgens supplement deficiencies, while antagonists block their effects in cancers. Insulin lowers blood glucose in diabetes. Levothyroxine treats hypothyroidism, while antithyroid drugs manage hyperthyroidism.

Understanding medication classifications allows systematic assessment of indications, mechanisms of action, potential adverse effects, interactions and contraindications to guide clinical pharmacotherapy decision making.

Prescription Abbreviations

Prescription writing utilizes many abbreviations and shorthand symbols to efficiently communicate medication instructions. Fluency with these notations helps ensure accurate prescription interpretation and dispensing. We will overview common abbreviations for doses, routes, frequencies, durations and special instructions.

Dose abbreviations include:

- mg - milligram
- g - gram
- mcg - microgram
- IU - International Units
- mEq - milliequivalent

Routes of administration include:

- PO - by mouth/orally
- IV - intravenous
- IM - intramuscular
- SQ - subcutaneous
- PR - rectal
- TOP - topical

- INH - inhalation
- SL - sublingual

Frequencies or timing abbreviations include:

- qAM - every morning
- qPM - every evening
- q4-6h - every 4 to 6 hours
- qid - four times daily
- tid - three times daily
- bid - twice daily
- qod - every other day
- hs - at bedtime

Duration abbreviations include:

- d - day
- wk - week
- mo - month

Other common abbreviations include:

- NPO - nothing by mouth
- ad lib - freely as desired
- stat - immediately
- soln - solution
- susp - suspension
- ext - extended release
- c - with
- ac - before meals
- pc - after meals

Latin abbreviations used include:

- per os (PO) - by mouth
- quaque die (QD) - every day
- quaque hora (QH) - every hour

Prescription clarity prevents misunderstandings and errors that can harm patients. Double-checking abbreviations ensures accurate transcription and appropriate medication provision. The introduction and use of technology like e-prescribing, improves legibility but abbreviations remain a commonplace. Understanding the shorthand language of prescription writing is very essential for all involved in medication management processes.

Medication Administration Terms

Medication administration requires precise communication between the prescriber, pharmacist and patient. We will define key terminology pertaining to routes, dosage forms, delivery methods and compliance to optimize accurate dispensing and proper usage for intended therapeutic benefits.

Enteral routes deliver medications directly into the gastrointestinal tract. Oral medications include tablets, capsules, liquids and solutions swallowed through the mouth. Sublingual administration involves placing under the tongue. Medications given rectally require insertion into the anus and absorption through the rectal mucosa. Parenteral routes bypass the GI system delivering medications into the body through other means. For example, Intravenous (IV) infusion directly injects medication into the bloodstream, intramuscular (IM) injection delivers medication deep into muscle tissue and subcutaneous (SQ) injection deposits medication into the fatty layer between skin and muscle. Medication dosage forms include tablets, capsules, solutions, suspensions, creams, ointments, inhalers, transdermal patches, suppositories and injectables. Modified release options control the medication release rate such as delayed, extended and controlled.

Solutions usually contain a drug that has already ben dissolved. Suspensions however, have undissolved particles evenly distributed throughout a liquid. Emulsions are two immiscible liquids with one dispersed as droplets in the other. Elixirs are clear, sweetened hydroalcoholic oral liquid medications and syrups are concentrated aqueous viscous solutions. Aerosolized inhalers deliver medications directly to the respiratory airways. Metered dose inhalers dispense sprays in fixed amounts per activation. Dry powder inhalers rely on inspiratory effort to fluidize and deliver powdered drug formulations. Transdermal patches adhere to skin allowing absorption over time, ophthalmic drops and ointments apply medication to the eye, otic drops instill medication into the ear canal and topical creams and ointments apply to localized areas of skin and mucous membranes.

Compliance means the patient takes their medication as prescribed. Adherence denotes following the regimen through active self-management. Concordance emphasizes shared decision making between the provider and patient. Noncompliance puts the patients at risks of subtherapeutic dosing and treatment failure.

Mastering medication terminology transforms complex concepts into clear communication enabling optimal therapeutic outcomes.

CHAPTER 7

ADVANCED MEDICAL TERMINOLOGY

Genetic Disorders and Terms

Understanding human genetics and associated terminology provides context for approaching genetic diseases. We will overview fundamental genetic principles and define key terms relevant to inherited conditions, mutations, chromosomal abnormalities and molecular testing.

The human DNA comprises of over 20,000 genes encoded on 23 chromosome pairs - 22 autosomal chromosomes and the sex chromosomes X and Y. Genes act as instructions to make specific proteins performing essential biological functions. Gene mutations alter the DNA sequence, potentially impairing protein synthesis and function. Genetic disorders arise from abnormalities inherited through germline mutations or acquired later in life through somatic mutations. Single gene disorders reflect mutations in one gene while multifactorial inheritance involves interplay between multiple genes and environmental factors.

Autosomal dominant disorders manifest when one mutated copy of a gene is present. Examples include neurofibromatosis, Marfan syndrome and familial hypercholesterolemia. Autosomal recessive conditions require two mutated copies, exemplified by cystic fibrosis and sickle cell disease. X-linked disorders like hemophilia mainly affect males who have the aberrant gene on their single X chromosome. Chromosomal abnormalities involve extra, missing or rearranged chromosomal material. Down syndrome results from trisomy 21, three copies of chromosome 21 instead of two. Monosomy on the other hand, refers to missing a chromosome. Translocations swap chromosome sections between nonhomologous chromosomes.

Cytogenetic analysis detects chromosomal abnormalities, karyotyping visualizes chromosomes stained and arranged by size and fluorescence in situ hybridization (FISH) uses fluorescent probes binding to specific sequences. Microarray testing identifies gains or losses of chromosomal material. Molecular genetic testing identifies disease-causing mutations in specific genes. Targeted tests analyze specified genes correlated to a suspected disorder, panel testing examines multiple related genes and whole exome and genome sequencing scan the protein coding regions or entire genome.

Understanding fundamental genetic principles and terminology related to inherited conditions provides context for recognizing at-risk patients, pursuing appropriate diagnostic testing, and providing genetic counseling around results and recurrence risks.

Terms in Surgical Procedures

Mastering the language of surgery enables seamless team communication and precision documentation to optimize patient outcomes. We will define key terminology related to surgical instrumentation, incisions, dissections, resections, repairs, implants, closures and postoperative considerations.

Incisions utilizing scalpels or electrosurgical units, provide access to surgical sites. Exploring the area aids visualization and palpation of anatomy. Retractors expose target structures while minimizing trauma and meticulous hemostasis with cautery, clips and suture ligation facilitates dissection. Dissecting through tissue planes requires skillful use of instruments like dissectors, scissors, and needle drivers along with manual traction and countertraction. Careful blunt dissection preserves the nerves and vessels. Performing a sharp dissection may be faster but provides the risk of damage. Excising diseased tissue for biopsy or resecting tumors and organs utilizes scalpels, scissors, electrosurgery and staplers. Wide local excision ensures negative margins. Sentinel lymph node mapping guides selective node dissections. Repairing structures may involve suturing healthy ends together after resection. Anastomoses restore gastrointestinal continuity, bypasses route around obstructions using native vessels or grafts and ostomies exteriorize the bowel through the abdominal wall.

Implants provide function or support after tissue removal and mesh reinforces soft tissue reconstruction. Prosthetics replace joints, valves, or blood vessels, stents scaffold open structures and hardware like plates, screws and rods stabilize fractures. Closure begins with irrigating and achieving hemostasis. Deep sutures provide strength while subcuticular stitches minimize scarring. Staples allow rapid skin closure, drains prevent fluid accumulation and steristrips, adhesives and dressings protect incisions.

Postoperative orders cover pain control, ambulation timing, diet advancement, wound care and monitoring for complications like bleeding, infections and thromboembolic events. Outpatient follow up continues recovery surveillance.

Fluency with surgical terminology transforms abstract concepts into clear communication to guide treatment decision making, seamless workflow and accurate documentation.

Innovations in Medical Technology

Medical technology continues advancing at a remarkable pace, providing clinicians with powerful new diagnostic and therapeutic tools. We will overview key innovations transforming modern healthcare across medical specialties.

Medical imaging evolves rapidly. Functional MRI visualizes brain activity, high resolution CT enters the nano scale, 3D and 4D ultrasound enrich obstetric evaluation and Molecular imaging identifies biochemical processes using radioactive tracers. Augmented reality is also integrated into ultrasound guidance and surgical navigation.

Robotics has revolutionized surgery. Robotic platforms provide motion scaling, tremor reduction and superior visualization benefiting complex procedures. Computer aided navigation improves surgical accuracy, simulators facilitate training and exoskeletons enhance rehabilitation. Making use of autonomous robots support disinfection and transportation roles. Genomics expands from research into clinical application. Next generation sequencing enables high throughput analysis. Pharmacogenomics guide personalized medicine, molecular diagnostics identify infections and biomarkers while gene editing therapies show curative potential. However, some ethical concerns still remain.

Mobile health makes uses of technological devices such smartphones and wearables. These devices track exercise, sleep, vital signs and more providing patients with lifestyle and health insights. Telemedicine expands access to providers via video visits and remote monitoring enables prompter intervention outside hospitals. These hoever still pose cybersecurity risks.

Point of care testing decentralizes diagnostics. Handheld devices analyze blood gases, cardiac markers, coagulation and more at the bedside. Smartphone attachments permit infection testing and chips enable nucleic acid analysis. Rapid results aid prompt treatment decisions.

These innovations have improved patient outcomes but require ongoing appraisal of clinical value, cost-effectiveness and ethical dimensions. Embracing change driven by human creativity and technology reflects medicine's timeless calling to tirelessly serve suffering humanity.

Interpreting Complex Case Reports

Case reports detail clinical presentations, diagnostic workups, therapeutic interventions, and outcomes of individual patient encounters. While anecdotal, they provide valuable educational insights that enrich medical knowledge. We will overview interpreting key elements and synthesizing clinical pearls from complex case reports.

The patient background sets the context, describing demographics, comorbidities and medications establishing the clinical milieu. A complete but focused review of symptoms clarifies the issues needing addressed. Pertinent history questions uncover social, family, occupational, environmental and habitual factors enabling a holistic perspective. The physical exam looks beyond the obvious, making god use of inspection, palpation, percussion and auscultation to recognize subtle findings informing differential diagnoses. Investigations like labs, imaging, pathology, and procedures generate objective data to support clinical decision making.

Complex reasoning connects findings to filter possibilities and focus the differential upon the most likely explanatory diagnoses. Subspecialty input, literature review and diagnostic testing help distinguish among rivals to reach the final diagnosis. Establishing causation requires eliminating plausible alternatives.

The discussion reviews the key factors supporting the final diagnosis. Teaching points highlight pearls distinguishing the presentation from mimics. Management principles flow logically from the diagnosis, addressing both the immediate issues and long term implications. Outcomes demonstrate the validity of the approach in resolving or controlling the clinical problems. Despite the uniqueness of each patient, generalizable lessons emerge from every case. Recognizing critical patterns among details and distilling clinical reasoning help transfer knowledge between presentations. Building a conceptual framework enables meaningful application of isolated facts through synthesis into broader clinical principles. Thoughtful interpretation of complex case reports provides a catalyst for mastering medical decision making. Discerning the clinical pearls within each narrative text cultivates discernment and wisdom benefitting all future patients.

CHAPTER 8

KEY TERMS

The Digestive System

1. **Esophagus** - The muscular tube that conveys food from the throat to the stomach.

2. **Stomach** - A hollow organ in which the major part of the digestion of food occurs.

3. **Small Intestine** - The part of the intestine where most of the end absorption of nutrients occurs; it includes the duodenum, jejunum, and ileum.

4. **Large Intestine** - The last part of the digestive system, where water is absorbed from the food and the remaining material is excreted as feces.

5. **Liver** - A large glandular organ that processes and detoxifies chemicals, and secretes bile.

6. **Gallbladder** - A small organ that stores bile produced by the liver and releases it into the small intestine.

7. **Pancreas** - An organ that produces enzymes for digestion and hormones for glucose regulation.

8. **Appendix** - A small tube attached to the large intestine, which has no function in digestion.

9. **Anus** - The opening at the end of the digestive tract through which feces exit the body.

10. **Bile** - A digestive fluid produced by the liver and stored in the gallbladder that helps in the digestion of fats.

11. **Digestive Enzymes** - Proteins that speed up the breakdown of food into nutrients.

12. **Gastrointestinal Tract (GI Tract)** - The series of hollow organs joined in a long, twisting tube from the mouth to the anus.

13. **Peristalsis** - The series of wave-like muscle contractions that move food through the digestive tract.

14. **Mucosa** - The lining of the GI tract that secretes mucus, digestive enzymes, and hormones.

15. **Submucosa** - A layer of tissue under the mucosa, containing blood vessels, nerves, and glands.

16. **Pylorus** - The part of the stomach that connects to the small intestine.

17. **Villi** - Small, finger-like projections that increase the surface area of the intestinal lining to help absorb nutrients.

18. **Chyme** - The pulpy acidic fluid that passes from the stomach to the small intestine, consisting of gastric juices and partly digested food.

19. **Colon** - A major part of the large intestine, absorbing water and salts from material that has not been digested as food, and is thus a key part of the process of excretion.

20. **Duodenum** - The first part of the small intestine immediately beyond the stomach, leading to the jejunum.

21. **Jejunum** - The middle section of the small intestine between the duodenum and ileum.

22. **Ileum** - The last and longest portion of the small intestine.

23. **Sphincter** - A ring of muscle that contracts to close an opening; several are found within the digestive system, such as the pyloric sphincter between the stomach and duodenum.

24. **Salivary Glands** - Glands located around the mouth that secrete saliva to initiate the digestion of carbohydrates.

25. **Fundus** - The upper part of the stomach, which serves as a temporary storage area.

26. **Gastric Juice** - A mixture of hydrochloric acid, digestive enzymes, and other substances produced by the stomach to digest food.

27. **Hepatic Duct** - The duct that conveys bile from the liver into the common bile duct.

28. **Cystic Duct** - The duct that conveys bile to and from the gallbladder.

29. **Common Bile Duct** - The duct formed by the union of the cystic duct and hepatic duct that carries bile into the small intestine.

30. **Mesentery** - A fold of membrane that attaches the intestine to the abdominal wall and holds it in place.

31. **Rectum** - The final section of the large intestine, terminating at the anus.

32. **Feces** - Waste matter remaining after digestion and absorption, expelled through the anus.

33. **Flora** - The bacteria and other microorganisms that live in the digestive tract and assist with digestion.

34. **Gastroenterologist** - A doctor who specializes in the management of diseases of the gastrointestinal tract.

35. **Gastritis** - Inflammation of the stomach lining.

36. **Ulcer** - An open sore on an external or internal surface of the body, caused by a break in the skin or mucous membrane that fails to heal.

37. **Gastroesophageal Reflux Disease (GERD)** - A chronic condition where stomach contents flow back into the esophagus, causing symptoms and potential damage.

38. **Lactase** - An enzyme that breaks down lactose into glucose and galactose; important for digesting dairy products.

39. **Peptic Ulcer** - An ulcer in the lining of the stomach or the first part of the small intestine.

40. **Hepatitis** - Inflammation of the liver, often caused by viral infections, toxins, or autoimmune disease.

41. **Barrett's Esophagus** - A condition in which the lining of the esophagus is damaged by stomach acid and is changed to a lining similar to that of the stomach.

42. **Choledocholithiasis** - The presence of at least one gallstone in the common bile duct.

43. **Cholecystitis** - Inflammation of the gallbladder, often due to a gallstone blocking its duct.

44. **Diverticulitis** - Inflammation or infection of one or more diverticula in the colon.

45. **Dysphagia** - Difficulty or discomfort in swallowing, as a symptom of disease.

46. **Enteritis** - Inflammation of the intestine, especially the small intestine.

47. **Fistula** - An abnormal connection or passageway that forms between two organs or vessels that normally do not connect.

48. **Gastroenteritis** - Inflammation of the stomach and intestines, typically resulting from bacterial toxins or viral infection and causing vomiting and diarrhea.

49. **Hemorrhoid** - Swollen and inflamed veins in the rectum and anus that cause discomfort and bleeding.

50. **Ileostomy** - A surgical operation in which a piece of the ileum is diverted to an artificial opening in the abdominal wall.

51. **Inflammatory Bowel Disease (IBD)** - A group of inflammatory conditions of the colon and small intestine, including Crohn's disease and ulcerative colitis.

52. **Jaundice** - Yellowing of the skin and whites of the eyes resulting from an accumulation of bilirubin in the blood; commonly associated with liver or bile duct dysfunction.

53. **Malabsorption** - A condition in which the small intestine does not absorb nutrients effectively.

54. **Nausea** - A feeling of sickness with an inclination to vomit.

55. **Pancreatitis** - Inflammation of the pancreas.

56. **Polyp** - A small growth, typically benign and with a stalk, protruding from a mucous membrane.

57. **Portal Hypertension** - High blood pressure in the portal venous system, which can lead to serious complications.

58. **Proctitis** - Inflammation of the lining of the rectum.

59. **Sigmoidoscopy** - A medical examination of the large intestine from the rectum through the nearest part of the colon, the sigmoid colon, using a device called a sigmoidoscope.

60. **Steatorrhea** - The presence of excess fat in feces, which can be indicative of digestive problems.

61. **Volvulus** - A condition in which a loop of intestine twists around itself and the mesentery that supports it, causing a bowel obstruction.

62. **Zollinger-Ellison Syndrome** - A condition in which one or more tumors form in the pancreas or the upper part of the small intestine, causing the stomach to produce too much acid, leading to peptic ulcers.

63. **Achalasia** - A disorder in which the esophagus has trouble moving food down into the stomach due to the lower esophageal sphincter being unable to relax.

64. **Ascites** - The accumulation of fluid in the peritoneal cavity, causing abdominal swelling; often due to cirrhosis of the liver.

65. **Bowel Obstruction** - A blockage that prevents food or liquid from passing through the small or large intestine.

66. **Celiac Disease** - An autoimmune disorder where the ingestion of gluten leads to damage in the small intestine.

67. **Colonoscopy** - A procedure that allows an examination of the entire colon using a flexible, camera-equipped tube.

68. **Crohn's Disease** - A type of inflammatory bowel disease (IBD) that may affect any part of the gastrointestinal tract from mouth to anus.

69. **Dyspepsia** - Indigestion or an upset stomach, characterized by abdominal pain, bloating, and sometimes nausea or vomiting.

70. **Endoscopy** - A procedure in which a long, flexible tube with a camera is used to view the digestive tract or other internal structures.

71. **Esophageal Varices** - Abnormally enlarged veins in the lower part of the esophagus, often associated with serious liver diseases.

72. **Gastroparesis** - A condition that affects the stomach muscles and prevents proper stomach emptying.

73. **Hepatomegaly** - Enlarged liver that can be due to various causes, including infections and tumors.

74. **Intussusception** - A medical condition in which a part of the intestine folds into the section next to it.

75. **Laparoscopy** - A surgical diagnostic procedure used to examine the organs inside the abdomen with only small incisions.

76. **Ostomy** - A surgical procedure creating an opening in the body for the discharge of body wastes.

77. **Peptic Ulcer Disease (PUD)** - An ulcerative disorder occurring in the stomach or the initial part of the small intestine.

78. **Peritonitis** - Inflammation of the peritoneum, often due to infection from a rupture or leakage in the abdominal area.

79. **Stoma** - An artificial opening created during an ostomy that allows for the passage of body wastes.

80. **Ulcerative Colitis** - A chronic inflammatory bowel disease that causes inflammation and ulcers in the colon and rectum.

81. **Whipple Procedure** - A complex surgical procedure usually performed to treat pancreatic or duodenal cancer, involving the removal of part of the pancreas, intestine, and sometimes other abdominal organs.

82. **Wilson's Disease** - A genetic disorder in which excess copper builds up in the body, often affecting the liver and leading to hepatic disease.

83. **Biliary Atresia** - A rare condition in infants where the bile ducts are abnormally narrow, blocked, or absent, leading to liver damage.

84. **Capsule Endoscopy** - A diagnostic procedure in which a small, pill-sized camera is swallowed to take images of the digestive tract, particularly useful for examining the small intestine.

85. **Cholangiography** - An imaging test used to look at the bile ducts to check for blockages or other abnormalities.

86. **Colitis** - Inflammation of the colon (large intestine), which can present with various symptoms such as diarrhea and abdominal pain.

87. **ERCP (Endoscopic Retrograde Cholangiopancreatography)** - A technique combining endoscopy and fluoroscopy to diagnose and treat conditions related to the bile ducts, gallbladder, and pancreas.

88. **Esophagectomy** - Surgical removal of all or part of the esophagus, often performed to treat esophageal cancer or severe esophageal disease.

89. **Gastric Bypass Surgery** - A type of weight-loss surgery that involves creating a small pouch from the stomach and connecting it directly to the small intestine.

90. **Gastrostomy** - A surgical procedure for inserting a tube through the abdomen into the stomach for feeding or drainage.

91. **Hematemesis** - Vomiting of blood, which can be a sign of serious gastrointestinal conditions such as ulcers or esophageal varices.

92. **Liver Biopsy** - A diagnostic procedure in which a small piece of liver tissue is removed for microscopic examination to diagnose liver diseases.

93. **Manometry** - A test commonly used to evaluate the function of the esophagus and bowel, measuring the pressure within these organs.

94. **Ménétrier's Disease** - A rare disorder characterized by overgrowth of the mucous membrane lining the stomach, leading to protein loss and enlarged stomach folds.

95. **Pancreaticoduodenectomy** - See Whipple Procedure (already mentioned as term 81).

96. **Pyloroplasty** - Surgical procedure to widen the opening of the pylorus, the exit area of the stomach, to allow contents to pass more freely into the small intestine.

97. **Sclerotherapy** - A treatment involving the injection of a solution into, for instance, hemorrhoids or esophageal varices to cause them to shrink.

98. **Total Parenteral Nutrition (TPN)** - Feeding a person intravenously, bypassing the usual process of eating and digestion. The person receives nutritional formulas that contain nutrients such as glucose, salts, amino acids, lipids, and added vitamins and dietary minerals.

99. **Transjugular Intrahepatic Portosystemic Shunt (TIPS)** - A procedure that creates a pathway within the liver for blood to flow easier to reduce high blood pressure in the veins of the stomach, esophagus, intestines, and liver.

100. **Zenker's Diverticulum** - A pouch that can form at the back of the throat, often causing difficulty swallowing, coughing, and other symptoms.

101. **Anastomosis** - A surgical connection between two structures. It is commonly used in gastrointestinal surgery to reconnect parts of the intestine or other hollow structures.

102. **Antrectomy** - Surgical removal of the antrum (the lower portion of the stomach), which is often performed to help reduce acid secretion and treat ulcers.

103. **Bezoar** - A mass found trapped in the gastrointestinal system, usually made up of hair or fiber, that the stomach cannot digest.

104. **Colonic Polypectomy** - The removal of polyps from the inside lining of the colon, typically performed during a colonoscopy.

105. **Dilatation and Curettage (D&C)** - Although more commonly associated with gynecological procedures, in the context of the digestive tract, dilatation can refer to the widening of a narrowed area in the esophagus, stomach, or intestines.

106. **Esophageal Stenting** - Placement of a stent (a tube) to keep the esophagus open in cases of obstruction or narrowing.

107. **Fecal Transplant** - A procedure where fecal bacteria from a healthy donor are transplanted to a patient's gastrointestinal tract for the treatment of certain conditions, such as Clostridium difficile infection.

108. **Gastric Electrical Stimulation** - A treatment method that involves sending mild electrical pulses to the stomach to help control nausea and vomiting for those with gastroparesis.

109. **Heller Myotomy** - A surgical procedure to cut the muscles at the lower end of the esophageal sphincter to relieve difficulty swallowing, typically due to achalasia.

110. **Intragastric Balloon** - A weight loss treatment that involves inserting a balloon into the stomach and then filling it with saline solution to help decrease food intake.

The Cardiovascular System

1. **Aorta** - The main artery that supplies oxygenated blood to the circulatory system.

2. **Aortic Stenosis** - Narrowing of the aorta, impeding blood flow from the heart.

3. **Arrhythmia** - Irregular heartbeat, either too fast or too slow.

4. **Arteriole** - Small branch of an artery leading into capillaries.

5. **Arteriosclerosis** - Thickening, hardening, and loss of elasticity of artery walls.

6. **Atherosclerosis** - Buildup of fats, cholesterol, and other substances in and on the artery walls.

7. **Atrial Fibrillation** - A common type of arrhythmia characterized by rapid and irregular beating of the atria.

8. **Bradycardia** - Abnormally slow heart rate.

9. **Capillary** - Smallest blood vessels where oxygen and nutrients are exchanged with tissues.

10. **Cardiac Arrest** - Sudden, unexpected loss of heart function, breathing, and consciousness.

11. **Cardiac Catheterization** - A procedure used to diagnose and treat cardiovascular conditions.

12. **Cardiac Output** - The volume of blood the heart pumps per minute.

13. **Cardiomyopathy** - Disease of the heart muscle that makes it harder for the heart to pump blood.

14. **Cardioversion** - A medical procedure that restores a normal heart rhythm in people with certain types of abnormal heartbeats.

15. **Carotid Artery** - Major blood vessels in the neck that supply blood to the brain, neck, and face.

16. **Cholesterol** - A type of fat, necessary for the body but too much can lead to health issues.

17. **Congenital Heart Disease** - Anomalies of the heart present from birth.

18. **Coronary Arteries** - Arteries that supply blood to the heart muscle.

19. **Coronary Artery Disease (CAD)** - Disease caused by the buildup of plaque resulting in the arteries narrowing or being blocked.

20. **Defibrillation** - A treatment for life-threatening cardiac dysrhythmias, usually ventricular fibrillation.

21. **Diastole** - Part of the cardiac cycle when the heart refills with blood.

22. **Echocardiogram** - A sonogram of the heart.

23. **Edema** - Swelling caused by excess fluid trapped in the body's tissues, often in the legs or arms.

24. **Electrocardiogram (ECG or EKG)** - A test that records the electrical activity of the heart.

25. **Endocarditis** - Inflammation of the inner layer of the heart, usually the valves.

26. **Fibrillation** - Rapid, irregular, and unsynchronized contraction of muscle fibers.

27. **Heart Attack (Myocardial Infarction)** - A blockage of blood flow to the heart muscle.

28. **Heart Failure** - A condition in which the heart is unable to pump sufficiently to maintain blood flow to meet the body's needs.

29. **Hemangioma** - A benign tumor of blood vessels, often appearing as a birthmark.

30. **Hemoglobin** - A protein in red blood cells that carries oxygen throughout the body.

31. **Hypertension** - High blood pressure, a state where blood pressure in the arteries is persistently elevated.

32. **Hypotension** - Abnormally low blood pressure.

33. **Ischemia** - An inadequate blood supply to an organ or part of the body, especially the heart muscles.

34. **Mitral Regurgitation** - A disorder in which the mitral valve does not close properly when the heart pumps out blood.

35. **Mitral Valve Prolapse** - A condition in which the two valve flaps of the mitral valve do not close smoothly or evenly, but bulge upward into the atrium.

36. **Murmur** - An unusual sound heard between heartbeats, sometimes sounding like a whooshing or swishing noise.

37. **Myocardium** - The muscular tissue of the heart.

38. **Pacemaker** - A device that regulates the heartbeat.

39. **Palpitation** - A noticeably rapid, strong, or irregular heartbeat due to agitation, exertion, or illness.

40. **Pericarditis** - Inflammation of the pericardium, the fluid-filled sac that surrounds the heart.

41. **Peripheral Arterial Disease (PAD)** - A condition where arteries are narrowed, reducing blood flow to the limbs.

42. **Phlebitis** - Inflammation of a vein.

43. **Plaque** - A substance that accumulates on the inner lining of an artery, composed of fat, cholesterol, calcium, and other materials found in the blood.

44. **Pulmonary Artery** - The artery carrying blood from the right ventricle of the heart to the lungs for oxygenation.

45. **Pulmonary Edema** - Accumulation of fluid in the lungs, often caused by heart failure.

46. **Pulmonary Embolism** - A blockage in one of the pulmonary arteries in the lungs usually caused by blood clots that travel to the lungs from the legs or other parts of the body.

47. **Pulmonary Vein** - A vein carrying oxygenated blood from the lungs to the left atrium of the heart.

48. **Pulse** - A rhythmic throbbing of the arteries as blood is propelled through them, typically felt in the wrists or neck.

49. **Saphenous Vein** - A large vein running along the length of the leg; often used for grafts in coronary artery bypass surgery.

50. **Septum** - The wall dividing the right and left sides of the heart.

51. **Sinoatrial Node** - The heart's natural pacemaker, which controls the heart rate by generating electrical impulses.

52. **Stenosis** - The abnormal narrowing of a passage in the body, such as a blood vessel or heart valve.

53. **Stent** - A tube inserted into a blocked passageway (often a coronary artery) to keep it open.

54. **Stroke** - A condition where poor blood flow to the brain results in cell death.

55. **Systole** - The phase of the heartbeat when the heart muscle contracts and pumps blood from the chambers into the arteries.

56. **Tachycardia** - An abnormally fast heart rate.

57. **Thrombosis** - Formation of a blood clot inside a blood vessel, obstructing the flow of blood through the circulatory system.

58. **Tricuspid Valve** - A valve that is situated at the opening of the right atrium of the heart into the right ventricle and consists of three triangular membranous flaps.

59. **Varicose Veins** - Veins that have become enlarged and twisted, most commonly appearing in the legs and feet.

60. **Vascular** - Relating to the body's blood vessels.

61. **Vasculitis** - Inflammation of the blood vessels that can cause changes in the blood vessel walls.

62. **Vasoconstriction** - The narrowing of blood vessels, which increases blood pressure.

63. **Vasodilation** - The widening of blood vessels, which decreases blood pressure.

64. **Vein** - A blood vessel that carries blood towards the heart.

65. **Vena Cava** - The two large veins (superior and inferior) that carry deoxygenated blood from the body into the heart.

66. **Venous Thromboembolism (VTE)** - A condition in which a blood clot forms most commonly in the deep veins of the leg and can travel in the circulation, lodging in the lungs, heart, or other area.

67. **Ventricular Fibrillation** - A severely abnormal heart rhythm that is life-threatening.

68. **Ventricular Septal Defect** - A hole in the heart's ventricular septum that causes blood to pass from the left to the right side of the heart.

69. **Ventricular Tachycardia** - A type of regular and fast heart rate that arises from improper electrical activity in the ventricles of the heart.

70. **Angioplasty** - A procedure to restore blood flow through the artery.

71. **Beta Blocker** - A medication that reduces blood pressure.

72. **Calcium Channel Blocker** - A type of medication that is typically used to manage high blood pressure.

73. **Cardiogenic Shock** - A condition where the heart suddenly can't pump enough blood to meet the body's needs.

74. **Diuretic** - A type of drug that increases the excretion of water from the body, commonly used to treat high blood pressure.

75. **Ejection Fraction** - Measurement of the percentage of blood leaving the heart each time it contracts.

76. **Heart Valve** - A flap in the heart that maintains blood flow in one direction through the heart.

77. **Inotrope** - A medication that alters the force or energy of heart contractions.

78. **Lipid Profile** - A blood test used to measure the amount of cholesterol and fats in the blood.

79. **Nitrate** - A medication that helps dilate blood vessels to prevent or reduce the intensity of chest pain.

80. **Orthostatic Hypotension** - A form of low blood pressure that happens when standing up from a sitting or lying position.

81. **Pericardiocentesis** - A procedure to remove fluid from the sac surrounding the heart.

82. **Peripheral Vascular Disease (PVD)** - Blood circulation disorder that causes the blood vessels outside of the heart and brain to narrow, block, or spasm.

83. **Petechiae** - Small red or purple spots caused by bleeding into the skin.

84. **Pulmonary Hypertension** - High blood pressure in the arteries to the lungs.

85. **Restenosis** - The re-narrowing of an artery after it has been treated to remove a blockage.

86. **Rheumatic Heart Disease** - Damage to the heart valves caused by rheumatic fever, which is caused by streptococcal bacteria.

87. **Sinus Rhythm** - The normal heartbeat rhythm, originating from the sinoatrial node.

88. **Sphygmomanometer** - An instrument for measuring blood pressure.

89. **Stress Test** - A test that measures the heart's ability to respond to external stress in a controlled clinical environment.

90. **Syncope** - Temporary loss of consciousness caused by a fall in blood pressure.

91. **Thrombectomy** - Surgical removal of a blood clot from a blood vessel.

92. **Thrombolysis** - The breakdown of blood clots by medications.

93. **Transesophageal Echocardiogram (TEE)** - An ultrasound imaging test that uses sound waves to create pictures of the heart via the esophagus.

94. **Triglycerides** - A type of fat (lipid) found in your blood.

95. **Ventriculography** - A test used to assess the heart's ability to pump blood and visualize the motion of the heart's walls.

96. **Venule** - A small vein that collects blood from capillaries and delivers it to larger veins.

97. **Viscosity** - A measure of the thickness and stickiness of an individual's blood.

98. **Vital Signs** - Clinical measurements, specifically pulse rate, temperature, respiration rate, and blood pressure, that indicate the state of a patient's essential body functions.

99. **Vascular Surgery** - Surgery performed to treat vascular diseases, which can involve the blood vessels, arteries, veins, or capillaries.

100. **Ventricular Assist Device (VAD)** - A mechanical pump used to support heart function and blood flow in individuals with weakened hearts.

101. **Waveform Analysis** - In cardiology, a method used to study the shape, amplitude, and features of waves seen in electrocardiogram readings.

102. **Window Operation** - A surgical procedure in which a window is created in the pericardium to relieve pressure from accumulated fluid.

103. **Xanthelasma** - A condition in which fat builds up under the surface of the skin, usually around the eyes, and can be indicative of high cholesterol levels.

104. **Yield Pressure** - The pressure at which a blood vessel will start to deform.

105. **Zollinger-Ellison Syndrome** - A condition caused by tumors that lead to excessive production of stomach acid, which can cause ulcers and affect gastrointestinal function, secondary impacting the cardiovascular system through stress and complication management.

106. **Epicardium** - The outer layer of the heart wall.

107. **Myocardial Infraction** - Commonly known as a heart attack, involving the interruption of blood supply to a part of the heart.

108. **Endothelium** - The inner lining of blood vessels.

109. **Blood Pool Imaging** - A nuclear medicine procedure used to evaluate the function and structure of the heart chambers.

110. **Angiogenesis** - The formation of new blood vessels.

111. **Blood Culture** - A test that is done to find an infection in the blood.

112. **Cardiac Enzyme Test** - Blood tests performed to determine the presence of cardiac enzymes, indicating heart muscle damage.

113. **Doppler Ultrasound** - A non-invasive test that can be used to estimate the blood flow through blood vessels.

114.   **Excisional Biopsy** - The removal of tissue from the body for examination, often used to diagnose diseases.

115.   **Heart Biopsy** - Taking a small piece of heart tissue for diagnostic purposes.

The Respiratory System

1. **Alveoli** - Tiny sacs within the lungs where gas exchange occurs.

2. **Bronchi** - The main passageways directly branching from the trachea into the lungs.

3. **Bronchioles** - Smaller branches of the bronchi that lead air to the alveoli.

4. **Cilia** - Microscopic hair-like structures lining the respiratory tract that move mucus out of the lungs.

5. **Diaphragm** - The primary muscle used in the process of breathing, located below the lungs.

6. **Epiglottis** - A flap of cartilage that covers the windpipe while swallowing to prevent inhalation of food.

7. **Glottis** - The part of the larynx consisting of the vocal cords and the slit-like opening between them.

8. **Larynx** - Also known as the voice box, it houses the vocal cords.

9. **Pharynx** - The membrane-lined cavity behind the nose and mouth, connecting them to the esophagus.

10. **Pleura** - A double-layered membrane surrounding each lung.

11. **Trachea** - Also known as the windpipe, it connects the pharynx and larynx to the lungs.

12. **Asthma** - A chronic inflammatory disease of the airways that causes periodic episodes of breathing difficulty.

13. **Bronchitis** - Inflammation of the bronchial tubes.

14. **COPD (Chronic Obstructive Pulmonary Disease)** - A chronic inflammatory lung disease that causes obstructed airflow from the lungs.

15. **Cystic Fibrosis** - A genetic disorder that affects the lungs and other organs, characterized by thick, sticky mucus.

16. **Emphysema** - A type of COPD that involves damage to the alveoli in the lungs.

17. **Hypoxia** - A condition in which the body or a region of the body is deprived of adequate oxygen supply.

18. **Pneumonia** - Infection that inflames the air sacs in one or both lungs, which may fill with fluid.

19. **Tuberculosis** - A serious infectious disease that mainly affects the lungs.

20. **Respiratory Rate** - The number of breaths a person takes per minute.

21. **Spirometry** - A common test used to assess how well your lungs work by measuring how much air you inhale, how much you exhale, and how quickly you exhale.

22. **Pulmonologist** - A doctor who specializes in the respiratory system.

23. **Nasal Passages** - The channels within the nose through which air flows.

24. **Mucus** - A sticky, slimy substance produced by the lining of the respiratory tract that traps dust, bacteria, and other debris.

25. **Sinuses** - Air-filled spaces in the skull that open into the nasal cavity.

26. **Apnea** - A temporary cessation of breathing, especially during sleep.

27. **Dyspnea** - Difficult or labored breathing.

28. **Tachypnea** - Abnormally rapid breathing.

29. **Bradypnea** - Abnormally slow breathing.

30. **Hyperventilation** - Breathing at an abnormally rapid rate, leading to decreased levels of carbon dioxide in the blood.

31. **Nebulizer** - A device that administers medication in the form of a mist inhaled into the lungs.

32. **Inhaler** - A device used to breathe in medication.

33. **Thorax** - The chest region that houses the heart and lungs.

34. **Intubation** - The insertion of a tube into the trachea to maintain an open airway.

35. **Ventilator** - A machine that provides mechanical ventilation by moving breathable air into and out of the lungs.

36. **Oximeter** - A device that measures the proportion of oxygenated hemoglobin in the blood.

37. **Pulse Oximetry** - A test used to measure the oxygen level (oxygen saturation) of the blood.

38. **Lobectomy** - Surgical removal of a lobe of the lung.

39. **Bronchoscopy** - A procedure that allows your doctor to examine your airway through a thin viewing instrument called a bronchoscope.

40. **Percussion** - A method used in physical examinations to determine the underlying structure of the chest.

41. **Auscultation** - Listening to the internal sounds of the body, typically using a stethoscope.

42. **Pleural Effusion** - Accumulation of fluid between the layers of tissue that line the lungs and the chest cavity.

43. **Pneumothorax** - Collapsed lung due to air in the pleural space.

44. **Pulmonary Edema** - Fluid accumulation in the air sacs of the lungs.

45. **Pulmonary Embolism** - A blockage in one of the pulmonary arteries in the lungs.

46. **Pulmonary Function Tests (PFTs)** - Tests that measure how well the lungs take in and release air and how well they move gases such as oxygen into the body's circulation.

47. **Respiratory Therapy** - Medical specialty focused on providing treatments that help improve lung function.

48. **Rhonchi** - Rattling sounds in the lungs that can be heard through a stethoscope and often sound like snoring.

49. **Stridor** - A harsh or grating sound caused by something that obstructs the airway.

50. **Thoracentesis** - A procedure to remove fluid or air from the pleural space.

51. **Tracheostomy** - A surgical procedure to create an opening through the neck into the trachea.

52. **V/Q Scan (Ventilation/Perfusion Scan)** - A medical scan that measures air and blood flow in the lungs.

53. **Wheezing** - A high-pitched whistling sound made while breathing.

54. **Bronchial Asthma** - A common type of asthma characterized by periodic wheezing, coughing, and shortness of breath.

55. **Chronic Bronchitis** - Long-term inflammation of the bronchi producing persistent cough that brings up mucus.

56. **Interstitial Lung Disease** - A group of lung disorders that cause progressive scarring of lung tissue.

57. **Laryngitis** - Inflammation of the larynx, often causing a hoarse voice or loss of voice.

58. **Lung Cancer** - A type of cancer that begins in the lungs.

59. **Nasal Conchae** - Curved bones that are responsible for filtering, warming, and humidifying the air we breathe.

60. **Oxygen Therapy** - The administration of oxygen as a medical intervention.

61. **Pulmonary Artery** - The artery carrying blood from the right ventricle of the heart to the lungs for oxygenation.

62. **Respirator** - A device designed to protect the wearer from inhaling harmful dusts, fumes, vapors, or gases.

63. **Sputum** - Mucus and other matter brought up from the lungs by coughing.

64. **Tracheitis** - Inflammation of the trachea.

65. **Upper Respiratory Infection (URI)** - An infection that affects the nasal passages and throat.

66. **Vocal Cords** - Bands of muscle located in the larynx that produce sound.

67. **Aspiration** - Breathing fluid, food, vomitus, or an object into the lungs.

68. **Capnography** - The monitoring of the concentration or partial pressure of carbon dioxide in the respiratory gases.

69. **Chest Tube** - A tube inserted into the pleural cavity to drain fluid, blood, or air and allow full expansion of the lungs.

70. **Expectorant** - Medication that helps bring up mucus and other material from the lungs, bronchi, and trachea.

71. **Hemothorax** - A collection of blood in the space between the chest wall and the lung (the pleural cavity).

72. **Inspiratory Capacity (IC)** - The amount of air that can be inhaled after the end of a normal expiration.

73. **Lung Compliance** - The measure of the lung's ability to stretch and expand.

74. **Pulmonary Hypertension** - Increased blood pressure within the pulmonary arteries.

75. **Respiratory Distress Syndrome** - A severe breathing problem that affects newborns and other individuals.

76. **Sleep Apnea** - A disorder characterized by pauses in breathing or periods of shallow breathing during sleep.

77. **Tidal Volume** - The amount of air which enters the lungs during normal inhalation at rest.

78. **Tracheal Stenosis** - The narrowing of the trachea.

79. **Tuberculin Skin Test** - A test used to determine if someone has developed an immune response to the bacterium that causes tuberculosis.

80. **Vital Capacity (VC)** - The maximum amount of air a person can expel from the lungs after a maximum inhalation.

81. **Bronchial Wash** - A procedure that involves washing out the bronchi with fluid to collect samples for examination.

82. **Lung Perfusion** - The circulation of blood through the lungs.

83. **Mantoux Test** - Another name for the tuberculin skin test.

84. **Nasal Septum** - The partition separating the two chambers

85. **Oropharynx** - The middle part of the pharynx that lies behind the oral cavity.

86. **Pleural Tap** - A procedure to remove fluid from the space between the lungs and the chest wall (pleural space).

87. **Pulmonary Alveolar Proteinosis** - A rare lung disease in which the alveoli fill up with proteinaceous material.

88. **Residual Volume** - The volume of air remaining in the lungs after a maximal exhalation.

89. **Thoracic Surgery** - Surgery performed on organs inside the thorax (the chest), primarily the heart and lungs.

90. **Tracheomalacia** - A condition where the tracheal cartilage is soft, leading to tracheal collapse especially when increased airflow is demanded.

91. **Bronchial Tubes** - Another term for the bronchi, the major airways leading into the lungs.

92. **Expiratory Reserve Volume** - The additional amount of air that can be forcibly exhaled after the expiration of a normal tidal volume.

93. **Inspiratory Reserve Volume** - The additional amount of air that can be forcibly inhaled after the inspiration of a normal tidal volume.

94. **Laryngopharynx** - The lower part of the pharynx just below the oropharyngeal opening into the larynx and esophagus.

95. **Mediastinoscopy** - A surgical procedure to examine the inside of the upper chest between and in front of the lungs (mediastinum).

96. **Nasopharynx** - The upper part of the pharynx, connecting with the nasal cavity above the soft palate.

97. **Pleural Rub** - A scratchy sound produced by pleural surfaces rubbing against each other.

98. **Pulmonary Lobectomy** - Surgical removal of a lobe of the lung.

99. **Spirometer** - An instrument used to measure the volume of air inhaled and exhaled by the lungs.

100. **Tracheal Intubation** - The placement of a flexible plastic tube into the trachea to maintain an open airway or to serve as a conduit through which to administer certain drugs.

101. **Bronchospasm** - A sudden constriction of the muscles in the walls of the bronchioles.

102. **Diffusion Capacity (DLCO)** - A test that measures how well gases such as oxygen are absorbed by the lungs.

103. **Expiratory Flow Rate** - The rate at which air can be expelled from the lungs.

104. **Hypercapnia** - Excessive carbon dioxide in the bloodstream, typically caused by inadequate respiration.

105. **Incentive Spirometry** - A medical device used to help patients improve the functioning of their lungs.

106. **Mucociliary Clearance** - The process of removing mucus and other materials from the lung by ciliary action.

107. **Pulmonary Rehabilitation** - A program of exercises and education to help patients with chronic respiratory disease.

108. **Respiratory Acidosis** - A condition arising when the lungs cannot remove all of the carbon dioxide the body produces.

109. **Segmentectomy** - Surgical removal of a segment of a lung.

110. **Total Lung Capacity** - The total volume of air contained in the lungs after the deepest possible breath.

111. **Bronchial Provocation Test** - A test to measure how sensitive the airways are by breathing in substances that cause narrowing of the airways.

112. **Carbon Dioxide (CO2) Retention** - A condition occurring when the lungs cannot expel carbon dioxide effectively.

113. **Lung Biopsy** - A procedure in which cells or tissues are removed from the lung for examination under a microscope.

114. **Paranasal Sinuses** - Air-filled spaces around the nasal cavity.

115. **Silicosis** - A lung disease caused by inhaling silica dust, leading to inflammation and scarring in the lungs.

The Nervous System

1. **Neuron** - The basic functional unit of the nervous system, responsible for transmitting information throughout the body.

2. **Axon** - The long, thin structure of a neuron that transmits electrical impulses away from the neuron's cell body.

3. **Dendrite** - The branched structures of a neuron that receive messages from other neurons.

4. **Synapse** - The junction between two nerve cells, where impulses pass by diffusion of a neurotransmitter.

5. **Neurotransmitter** - Chemicals that transmit signals across a synapse from one neuron to another.

6. **Myelin Sheath** - The fatty covering around axons that speeds up the transmission of nerve impulses.

7. **Cerebrum** - The largest part of the brain, responsible for voluntary muscular activity, vision, speech, taste, hearing, thought, and memory.

8. **Cerebellum** - A region of the brain that plays an important role in motor control and coordination.

9. **Brainstem** - The structure that connects the cerebrum of the brain to the spinal cord and mediates basic bodily functions.

10. **Spinal Cord** - The main pathway for information connecting the brain and peripheral nervous system.

11. **Peripheral Nervous System (PNS)** - The part of the nervous system that consists of the nerves and ganglia outside of the brain and spinal cord.

12. **Central Nervous System (CNS)** - Consists of the brain and spinal cord.

13. **Autonomic Nervous System (ANS)** - The part of the nervous system responsible for control of the bodily functions not consciously directed, such as breathing, the heartbeat, and digestive processes.

14. **Somatic Nervous System** - The part of the peripheral nervous system associated with the voluntary control of body movements via skeletal muscles.

15. **Motor Neurons** - Neurons that carry outgoing information from the brain and spinal cord to the muscles and glands.

16. **Sensory Neurons** - Neurons that carry incoming information from the sensory receptors to the brain and spinal cord.

17. **Interneurons** - Neurons that transmit impulses between other neurons, especially as part of reflex arcs.

18. **Glia** - Cells in the nervous system that support, nourish, and protect neurons.

19. **Astrocyte** - A type of glial cell that transports water and salts from capillaries.

20. **Schwann Cells** - Specialized cells that myelinate the axons of the peripheral nervous system.

21. **Oligodendrocyte** - A type of glial cell in the CNS that produces the myelin sheath.

22. **Synaptic Cleft** - The gap at the synapse between neurons.

23. **Action Potential** - A neural impulse; a brief electrical charge that travels down an axon.

24. **Reflex Arc** - The neural path of a reflex.

25. **Meninges** - The three protective membranes that surround the brain and spinal cord.

26. **Cerebrospinal Fluid (CSF)** - The fluid in and around the brain and spinal cord.

27. **Blood-Brain Barrier** - A mechanism that prevents certain molecule from entering the brain but allows others to cross.

28. **Cranial Nerves** - Twelve pairs of nerves that carry messages to and from the brain with regard to the head and neck.

29. **Spinal Nerves** - Thirty-one pairs of nerves arising from the spinal cord.

30. **Neuroplasticity** - The ability of the nervous system to change its activity in response to intrinsic or extrinsic stimuli by reorganizing its structure, functions, or connections.

31. **Neurogenesis** - The process of generating new neurons.

32. **Neuropathy** - Disease or dysfunction of one or more peripheral nerves, typically causing numbness or weakness.

33. **Epilepsy** - A neurological disorder marked by sudden recurrent episodes of sensory disturbance, loss of consciousness, or convulsions.

34. **Multiple Sclerosis (MS)** - A disease in which the immune system eats away at the protective covering of nerves.

35. **Parkinson's Disease** - A progressive disease of the nervous system marked by tremor, muscular rigidity, and slow, imprecise movement.

36. **Alzheimer's Disease** - A progressive neurodegenerative disease characterized by memory loss, language deterioration, and impaired ability to mentally manipulate visual information.

37. **Huntington's Disease** - A hereditary disease marked by degeneration of the brain cells and causing chorea and progressive dementia.

38. **Amyotrophic Lateral Sclerosis (ALS)** - A progressive neurodegenerative disease that affects nerve cells in the brain andthe spinal cord, leading to muscle weakness and atrophy.

39. **Neurology** - The branch of medicine dealing with disorders of the nervous system.

40. **Neuropsychology** - The study of the relationship between behavior, emotion, and cognition on the one hand, and brain function on the other.

41. **Neuralgia** - Intense, typically intermittent pain along the course of a nerve, especially in the head or face.

42. **Encephalopathy** - A broad term for any brain disease that alters brain function or structure.

43. **Migraine** - A neurological syndrome characterized by altered bodily perceptions, severe headaches, and nausea.

44. **Cerebral Palsy** - A congenital disorder of movement, muscle tone, or posture.

45. **Stroke** - A sudden disruption in blood supply to the brain, leading to neurological impairment.

46. **Transient Ischemic Attack (TIA)** - Often called a mini-stroke, a temporary period of symptoms similar to those of a stroke.

47. **Aphasia** - The impairment of language ability; this can affect speech, reading, and writing.

48. **Dysarthria** - A motor speech disorder resulting from neurological injury.

49. **Bell's Palsy** - A temporary paralysis of the facial muscles, causing drooping of one side of the face.

50. **Neural Tube Defects** - Birth defects of the brain, spine, or spinal cord.

51. **Meningitis** - An acute inflammation of the protective membranes covering the brain and spinal cord, known collectively as the meninges.

52. **Neurodegeneration** - The progressive loss of structure or function of neurons, including death of neurons.

53. **Demyelinating Disease** - Any condition that results in damage to the protective covering (myelin sheath) that surrounds nerve fibers in the brain, optic nerves, and spinal cord.

54. **Neuroendocrinology** - The study of the interaction between the nervous system and the endocrine system.

55. **Resting Potential** - The electrical charge across the cell membrane of a resting neuron.

56. **Depolarization** - A decrease in the electrical charge across a cell membrane; generally involves an influx of sodium ions.

57. **Repolarization** - The reestablishment of a polarized state in a neuron following depolarization.

58. **Hyperpolarization** - An increase in the membrane potential of a cell, relative to the normal resting potential.

59. **Nerve Conduction Study** - A diagnostic test that measures how quickly electrical signals move through your peripheral nerves.

60. **Electroencephalogram (EEG)** - A test that detects electrical activity in the brain using small, flat metal discs attached to the scalp.

61. **Computed Tomography (CT) of Brain** - A diagnostic imaging procedure that uses a combination of X-rays and computer technology to produce horizontal, or axial, images of the brain.

62. **Magnetic Resonance Imaging (MRI) of Brain** - An imaging test that uses powerful magnets and radio waves to create pictures of the brain and surrounding nerve tissues.

63. **Positron Emission Tomography (PET) Scan** - A test that uses a special type of camera and a tracer to look at organs in the body.

64. **Lumbar Puncture** - A procedure in which a needle is inserted into the spinal canal to collect cerebrospinal fluid for diagnostic testing.

65. **Cognitive Function** - A term referring to an individual's ability to process thoughts.

66. **Executive Functions** - Higher order thinking processes that include planning, organizing, inhibition, and decision-making.

67. **Sensory Processing Disorder** - A condition in which the brain has trouble receiving and responding to information that comes in through the senses.

68. **Neurotransmission** - The process by which signaling molecules called neurotransmitters are released by a neuron and bind to and activate the receptors of another neuron.

69. **Glioma** - A type of tumor that occurs in the brain and spinal cord.

70. **Neuromodulation** - The physiological process by which a given neuron uses one or more chemicals to regulate diverse populations of neurons.

71. **Neurotrophic Factors** - A family of proteins that are responsible for the growth and survival of developing neurons and the maintenance of mature neurons.

72. **Neuroanatomy** - The study of the structure and organization of the nervous system.

73. **Neuropathology** - The study of diseases of the nervous system tissue.

74. **Electromyography (EMG)** - A diagnostic procedure to assess the health of muscles and the nerve cells that control them (motor neurons).

75. **Nerve Growth Factor (NGF)** - A protein secreted by a neuron's target cell that promotes the survival and growth of the neuron.

76. **Nerve Block** - An injection of anesthetic to interrupt pain signals in a specific area of the body.

77. **Neuralgia** - Pain along the course of a nerve.

78. **Neuritis** - Inflammation of a nerve or the general inflammation of the peripheral nervous system.

79. **Neuroblastoma** - A cancer that develops from immature nerve cells found in several areas of the body.

80. **Neurocysticercosis** - A parasitic disease of the nervous system resulting from the ingestion of eggs from the pork tapeworm, Taenia solium.

81. **Neurofibroma** - A benign nerve sheath tumor in the peripheral nervous system.

82. **Neuromuscular Junction** - The synapse or junction of the motor neuron and the muscle it controls.

83. **Neuropathologist** - A specialist who studies diseases of the nerve tissue.

84. **Neuropharmacology** - The study of how drugs affect cellular function in the nervous system.

85. **Neurophysiology** - The study of the function of the nervous system.

86. **Neuroprotective** - Agents that are used to protect the central nervous system (CNS) from degeneration.

87. **Neurosurgery** - The surgical specialty concerned with the treatment of diseases and disorders of the brain, spinal cord, and peripheral nerves.

88. **Neurotoxin** - A toxin that specifically poisons nerve cells.

89. **Nociceptor** - A sensory receptor for painful stimuli.

90. **Optic Nerve** - The nerve that transmits visual information from the retina to the brain.

91. **Paresthesia** - An abnormal sensation, typically tingling or pricking ('pins and needles'), caused by pressure on or damage to peripheral nerves.

92. **Peripheral Neuropathy** - A result of damage to your peripheral nerves, often causing weakness, numbness, and pain, usually in your hands and feet.

93. **Radiculopathy** - A condition due to a compressed nerve in the spine that can cause pain, numbness, tingling, or weakness along the course of the nerve.

94. **Receptor** - A specialized cell or group of nerve endings that responds to sensory stimuli.

95. **Seizure** - A sudden surge of electrical activity in the brain, affecting how a person feels or acts.

96. **Sensory Cortex** - The part of the brain that receives and processes sensory information.

97. **Spina Bifida** - A neural tube defect characterized by incomplete closure of the backbone and membranes around the spinal cord.

98. **Spinal Decompression** - A type of therapy or surgical procedure that relieves pressure on a spinal nerve or the spinal cord.

99. **Subarachnoid Hemorrhage** - Bleeding in the area between the brain and the thin tissues covering the brain, typically caused by the rupture of an aneurysm.

100. **Synaptic Plasticity** - The ability of synapses to strengthen or weaken over time, in response to increases or decreases in their activity.

101. **Thalamus** - The brain's relay station for sensory and motor skills.

102. **Tremor** - Involuntary, rhythmic muscle contractions leading to shaking movements in one or more parts of the body.

103. **Vagus Nerve** - The tenth cranial nerve that innervates the digestive tract, heart, and other organs.

104. **Ventricles** - Hollow structures within the brain filled with cerebrospinal fluid.

105. **Vestibular System** - The sensory system that contributes to balance and spatial orientation.

106. **White Matter** - The paler tissue of the brain and spinal cord, consisting mainly of nerve fibers with their myelin sheaths.

107. **Wernicke's Area** - A region of the brain concerned with the comprehension of language, located in the cortex of the dominant temporal lobe.

108. **Acoustic Neuroma** - A noncancerous tumor that develops on the nerve that connects the ear to the brain.

109. **Basal Ganglia** - A group of structures linked to the thalamus in the base of the brain and involved in coordination of movement.

110. **Brain Mapping** - A set of neuroscience techniques used to create a map of the various brain areas and their functions.

111. **Cranial Electrotherapy Stimulation** - A form of neurostimulation that delivers a small, pulsed electric current across a person's head.

112. **Deep Brain Stimulation** - A neurosurgical procedure involving the implantation of a medical device called a neurostimulator, which sends electrical impulses to specific targets in the brain.

113. **Gamma Knife** - A type of radiation therapy used to treat abnormalities in the brain.

114. **Cerebral Edema** - Swelling of the brain caused by the accumulation of fluid in the brain tissue, which can result from various causes including traumatic injury, infection, or high altitude sickness.

115. **Cerebrospinal Fluid Analysis** - A diagnostic test involving the collection and examination of the fluid surrounding the brain and spinal cord, used to diagnose conditions affecting the central nervous system such as infections, bleeding, and multiple sclerosis.

The Visual System

1. **Acuity** - The clarity or sharpness of vision.

2. **Aqueous Humor** - The clear fluid filling the space in the front of the eyeball between the lens and the cornea.

3. **Astigmatism** - A condition in which the cornea is irregularly shaped, causing blurred vision.

4. **Bifocal** - Lenses containing two points of focus, usually for near and distance vision.

5. **Binocular Vision** - The ability to maintain visual focus on an object with both eyes, creating a single visual image.

6. **Blind Spot** - The point on the retina where the optic nerve exits; lacks photoreceptors and is insensitive to light.

7. **Cataract** - Clouding of the lens of the eye, causing impaired vision.

8. **Choroid** - The layer of blood vessels and connective tissue between the sclera and the retina of the eye.

9. **Cones** - Photoreceptor cells in the retina that are responsible for color vision.

10. **Conjunctiva** - The mucous membrane that covers the front of the eye and lines the inside of the eyelids.

11. **Cornea** - The transparent outer covering of the eye that covers the iris and pupil.

12. **Dilation** - Widening or enlargement of the pupil, controlled by muscles in the iris.

13. **Diplopia** - Double vision; the perception of two images from a single object.

14. **Drusen** - Tiny yellow or white accumulations of extracellular material that build up in the retina, commonly associated with aging.

15. **Fovea** - The central part of the macula that provides the sharpest vision.

16. **Fundus** - The interior surface of the eye opposite the lens, includes the retina, optic disc, and blood vessels.

17. **Glaucoma** - A group of eye conditions that damage the optic nerve, often caused by abnormally high pressure in the eye.

18. **Hyperopia** - Farsightedness; difficulty focusing on close objects.

19. **Iris** - The colored part of the eye, which controls the size of the pupil and amount of light that enters the eye.

20. **Keratitis** - Inflammation of the cornea.

21. **Lacrimal Glands** - Glands located in the upper outer region of the orbit that produce tears.

22. **Lens** - The transparent structure inside the eye that focuses light rays onto the retina.

23. **Macula** - A small central area in the retina that contains a high concentration of cones and is responsible for detailed central vision.

24. **Myopia** - Nearsightedness; difficulty focusing on distant objects.

25. **Nystagmus** - Involuntary rapid eye movements.

26. **Ocular** - Pertaining to the eye.

27. **Optic Chiasm** - The X-shaped structure formed at the point below the brain where the two optic nerves cross over each other.

28. **Optic Disc** - The region at the back of the eye where the optic nerve meets the retina.

29. **Optic Nerve** - The nerve that transmits visual information from the retina to the brain.

30. **Peripheral Vision** - The ability to see objects and movement outside of the direct line of vision.

31. **Photophobia** - Sensitivity to light.

32. **Photoreceptor Cells** - Cells in the retina that begin the process of converting light into vision. There are two types: rods and cones.

33. **Presbyopia** - The gradual loss of the eye's ability to focus on nearby objects, commonly associated with aging.

34. **Pupil** - The opening in the center of the iris through which light enters the eye.

35. **Refraction** - The bending of light as it passes through one object to another.

36. **Retina** - The light-sensitive layer of tissue at the back of the eye.

37. **Retinal Detachment** - A serious condition where the retina pulls away from the layer of blood vessels that provides it with oxygen and nutrients.

38. **Rods** - Photoreceptor cells in the retina that are sensitive to low light conditions.

39. **Sclera** - The white outer layer of the eyeball.

40. **Scotoma** - A partial loss of vision or a blind spot in an otherwise normal visual field.

41. **Slit Lamp** - A microscope used to examine the eye; especially the cornea, iris, and lens.

42. **Strabismus** - Misalignment of the eyes, commonly known as cross-eyed or wall-eyed.

43. **Tonometer** - An instrument used to measure the pressure inside the eye, commonly used in diagnosing glaucoma.

44. **Trabecular Meshwork** - A sponge-like tissue located around the base of the cornea, responsible for draining the aqueous humor from the eye.

45. **Uvea** - The middle layer of the eye that includes the iris, ciliary body, and choroid.

46. **Uveitis** - Inflammation of the uvea, potentially causing swelling and damage to the eye tissues.

47. **Vitreous Humor** - The clear gel that fills the space between the lens and the retina of the eyeball.

48. **Visual Acuity Test** - A common eye test to measure the smallest letters you can read on a standardized chart (Snellen chart) at a distance.

49. **Visual Cortex** - The part of the cerebral cortex responsible for processing visual information.

50. **Visual Field Test** - A test that measures all areas of eyesight, including peripheral vision.

51. **Xanthelasma** - Soft, cholesterol-filled plaques that appear on the eyelids.

52. **Zeiss Glands** - Sebaceous glands in the eyelids that help lubricate the eye.

53. **Zonules of Zinn** - A series of fibers connecting the ciliary body and lens of the eye, helping to hold the lens in place and adjust its shape during focusing.

54. **Anisocoria** - Condition where the pupils of the eyes are different sizes.

55. **Anterior Chamber** - The fluid-filled space inside the eye between the cornea and the iris.

56. **Blepharitis** - Inflammation of the eyelids, usually involving the part of the eyelid where eyelashes grow.

57. **Central Retinal Artery** - The artery that supplies oxygen-rich blood to the retina.

58. **Central Retinal Vein** - The vein that carries blood away from the retina.

59. **Color Blindness** - A condition where a person is unable to distinguish certain colors.

60. **Corneal Abrasion** - A scratch on the surface of the cornea.

61. **Corneal Transplant** - A surgical procedure to replace part of the cornea with corneal tissue from a donor.

62. **Cryotherapy for Retinopathy** - A treatment that uses extreme cold to destroy abnormal blood vessels in the retina.

63. **Dark Adaptation** - The process by which the eyes increase their sensitivity in low light.

64. **Diabetic Retinopathy** - Damage to the retinal blood vessels in a person with diabetes.

65. **Electroretinography** - A test to measure the electrical response of the eye's light-sensitive cells, called rods and cones.

66. **Enucleation** - The removal of the eye leaving the eye muscles and remaining orbital contents intact.

67. **Exophthalmos** - Bulging of the eye anteriorly out of the orbit.

68. **Fluorescein Angiography** - A medical procedure in which a fluorescent dye is injected into the bloodstream to highlight the blood vessels in the back of the eye.

69. **Gonioscopy** - An eye examination to look at the front part of your eye (anterior chamber) between the cornea and the iris.

70. **Heterochromia** - A condition in which the colored part of the eye (iris) is multicolored.

71. **Intraocular Lens (IOL)** - A synthetic lens implanted in the eye to replace a natural lens that has been removed, usually because of cataracts.

72. **Intraocular Pressure (IOP)** - The fluid pressure inside the eye.

73. **Iris Coloboma** - A keyhole-shaped defect of the iris.

74. **Keratoconus** - A progressive disease in which the cornea thins and begins to bulge into a cone-like shape.

75. **Laser Trabeculoplasty** - A laser treatment that helps fluid drain out of the eye, often used to treat glaucoma.

76. **Legal Blindness** - A condition of severely impaired vision; defined legally as vision that cannot be corrected to better than 20/200.

77. **Macular Edema** - Swelling or thickening of the macula, the part of the retina responsible for detailed, central vision.

78. **Macular Hole** - A small break in the macula, leading to vision loss.

79. **Macular Pucker** - Scar tissue that has formed on the eye's macula, located in the center of the light-sensitive retina.

80. **Night Blindness** - The inability to see well at night or in poor light.

81. **Ocular Prosthesis** - An artificial eye, typically used to replace an eye that has been removed for medical reasons.

82. **Ophthalmoscope** - An instrument used by doctors to examine the inside of the eye, including the retina and optic nerve.

83. **Optic Atrophy** - Damage to the optic nerve resulting in a degradation of vision.

84. **Optic Neuritis** - Inflammation of the optic nerve that can cause a sudden reduction of vision.

85. **Orthoptist** - A specialist who treats disorders of eye movements and problems related to how the eyes work together.

86. **Pachymetry** - The measurement of the thickness of the cornea.

87. **Panretinal Photocoagulation** - A type of laser surgery used primarily to treat proliferative diabetic retinopathy by reducing the oxygen demand of the retina.

88. **Patching** - Covering one eye to encourage the use of the other eye, typically used to treat amblyopia (lazy eye).

89. **Peripheral Iridotomy** - A laser treatment to make a small hole in the iris, helping fluid to flow to the front of the eye and reduce eye pressure.

90. **Phacoemulsification** - A modern cataract surgery method that uses ultrasonic waves to emulsify the cloudy lens before it's suctioned out.

91. **Photodynamic Therapy** - A treatment that involves light-sensitive medication and a light source to destroy abnormal blood vessels in the eye.

92. **Pigment Dispersion Syndrome** - A condition in which pigment granules that normally adhere to the back of the iris flake off into the clear fluid inside the eye.

93. **Pinguecula** - A yellowish, slightly raised thickening of the conjunctiva on the white part of the eye near the cornea.

94. **Pterygium** - A benign growth of the conjunctiva that can expand over the cornea, potentially impacting vision.

95. **Ptosis** - Drooping of the upper eyelid, which may cover all or part of the pupil and interfere with vision.

96. **Retinal Pigment Epithelium** - A layer of cells that nourishes the retinal cells and is essential for visual function.

97. **Retinoscopy** - A test to obtain an objective measurement of the refractive error of the eyes.

98. **Scleritis** - An inflammation of the sclera, the white outer layer of the eyeball, often linked to autoimmune disorders.

99. **Secondary Cataract** - A condition that can occur after cataract surgery; also called posterior capsule opacification.

100. **Slit-Lamp Examination** - A procedure that uses an intense line of light (a slit) to illuminate the cornea, iris, lens, and the space between the iris and cornea.

101. **Stereopsis** - The ability to perceive and understand three-dimensional space using both eyes.

102. **Trachoma** - A bacterial infection that affects the eyes and can cause chronic conjunctivitis and lead to blindness.

103. **Ultrasound Biomicroscopy** - A diagnostic imaging technique that uses high-frequency ultrasound to provide detailed images of the anterior segment of the eye.

104. **Visual Evoked Potential (VEP)** - A test that measures electrical activity in the brain in response to visual stimuli.

105. **Vitreoretinal Surgery** - Surgery used to treat disorders related to the retina and vitreous fluid, including retinal detachment.

106. **Vitritis** - Inflammation of the vitreous body in the eye, often due to infection or inflammatory diseases.

107. **Xerophthalmia** - A medical condition in which the eye fails to produce tears, often associated with vitamin A deficiency.

108.   **YAG Laser Capsulotomy** - A laser treatment used to clear vision after cataract surgery when part of the lens capsule remains cloudy.

109.   **Zeaxanthin** - A dietary carotenoid found in the retina, believed to contribute to eye health.

110.   **Zonular Fibers** - Fibers that connect the ciliary body and lens of the eye, helping to hold the lens in place and adjust its shape during focusing.

111.   **Aberration** - Distortion in vision typically resulting from irregularities in the cornea or lens of the eye.

112.   **Amblyopia** - Also known as lazy eye, a condition where the eye and brain do not work together properly resulting in decreased vision in an eye that otherwise typically appears normal.

113.   **Aniridia** - A rare congenital condition characterized by the absence of the iris, usually in both eyes.

114.   **Blepharospasm** - An abnormal, involuntary blinking or spasm of the eyelids.

115.   **Canthoplasty** - A surgical procedure aimed at modifying the lateral canthus (the outer corner where the upper and lower eyelids meet) to change the shape of the eye or improve its function. This can be done for both cosmetic reasons or to correct structural issues that affect eyelid function.

The Auditory System

1. **Acoustic Neuroma** - A benign tumor on the nerve that connects the ear to the brain.

2. **Audiogram** - A chart that records the results of a hearing test.

3. **Audiologist** - A healthcare professional specializing in identifying, diagnosing, treating, and monitoring disorders of the auditory and vestibular systems.

4. **Audiometry** - The measurement of hearing ability, including tests of hearing sensitivity and acuity.

5. **Aural Atresia** - A congenital absence or closure of the external auditory ear canal.

6. **Autoacoustic Emissions** - Sounds emitted by the inner ear when the cochlea is stimulated by sound.

7. **Bilateral Hearing Loss** - Hearing loss in both ears.

8. **Bone Conduction** - Transmission of sound through the bones of the skull to the inner ear.

9. **Cerumen** - Ear wax, a substance that protects the ear canal by trapping dirt and slowing the growth of bacteria.

10. **Cholesteatoma** - An abnormal skin growth in the middle ear behind the eardrum.

11. **Cochlea** - The spiral-shaped, fluid-filled inner ear structure that is responsible for hearing.

12. **Cochlear Implant** - A device that provides direct electrical stimulation to the auditory (hearing) nerve in the inner ear.

13. **Conductive Hearing Loss** - Hearing loss caused by an obstruction or damage to the outer or middle ear.

14. **Decibel (dB)** - A unit used to measure the intensity of a sound or the power level of an electrical signal by comparing it with a given level on a logarithmic scale.

15. **Dichotic Listening** - A test procedure used to investigate selective listening and the brain's ability to process different sounds in each ear.

16. **Ear Canal** - The tube that runs between the outer ear and the middle ear.

17. **Eardrum (Tympanic Membrane)** - A thin membrane that vibrates in response to sound waves and separates the outer ear from the middle ear.

18. **Endolymph** - The fluid contained within the membranous labyrinth of the inner ear.

19. **Eustachian Tube** - A canal that links the middle ear with the throat area and helps to equalize pressure in the middle ear.

20. **Hair Cells** - Sensory cells in the inner ear that are essential for hearing.

21. **Hearing Aid** - An electronic device worn in or behind the ear to amplify sound.

22. **Hyperacusis** - An increased sensitivity to normal environmental sounds.

23. **Impedance Audiometry** - A test that measures the resistance of the middle ear to sound conduction.

24. **Incus** - The anvil-shaped small bone or ossicle in the middle ear.

25. **Inner Ear** - The innermost part of the ear, containing the cochlea, vestibule, and semicircular canals.

26. **Labyrinthitis** - Inflammation of the inner ear or the nerves that connect the ear to the brain.

27. **Malleus** - The hammer-shaped small bone or ossicle in the middle ear.

28. **Meniere's Disease** - A disorder of the inner ear that can lead to dizzy spells (vertigo) and hearing loss.

29. **Middle Ear** - The air-filled central cavity of the ear behind the eardrum.

30. **Mixed Hearing Loss** - A combination of conductive and sensorineural hearing losses.

31. **Ossicles** - The three small bones in the middle ear (malleus, incus, and stapes) that transmit sound vibrations.

32. **Otitis Externa** - Inflammation of the outer ear canal, also known as swimmer's ear.

33. **Otitis Media** - Inflammation or infection of the middle ear.

34. **Otoacoustic Emission Testing (OAE)** - A test that measures an acoustic response produced by the inner ear when stimulated by sound.

35. **Otology** - The branch of medicine that focuses on the ears and their diseases.

36. **Otosclerosis** - An abnormal bone growth in the middle ear that causes hearing loss.

37. **Outer Ear** - The external portion of the ear, which includes the auricle and the ear canal.

38. **Perilymph** - The fluid that fills the space between the membranous labyrinth of the inner ear and the bone that encloses it.

39. **Pinna** - The visible part of the outer ear that collects sound and directs it into the auditory canal.

40. **Presbycusis** - Age-related hearing loss.

41. **Sensorineural Hearing Loss** - Hearing loss caused by damage to the sensory cells and/or nerve fibers of the inner ear or the auditory pathway to the brain.

42. **Stapedectomy** - A surgical procedure to replace the stapes bone in the middle ear with a prosthetic device.

43. **Stapes** - The stirrup-shaped small bone or ossicle in the middle ear, involved in the conduction of sound vibrations to the inner ear.

44. **Tinnitus** - The hearing of sound when no external sound is present, often described as ringing in the ears.

45. **Tympanogram** - A test that measures the movement of the eardrum in response to changes in air pressure.

46. **Tympanometry** - The examination of the middle ear by recording the movement of the eardrum through the variation of air pressure in the ear canal.

47. **Tympanoplasty** - Surgical repair of a perforated eardrum or defects of the middle ear.

48. **Vestibular System** - A complex system in the inner ear that contributes to balance and spatial orientation.

49. **Vestibulocochlear Nerve** - The eighth cranial nerve that carries auditory and balance information from the inner ear to the brain.

50. **Acoustic Reflex** - An involuntary muscle contraction in the middle ear in response to high-intensity sound stimuli.

51. **Auditory Brainstem Response (ABR)** - A test used to measure hearing sensitivity and the function of the auditory nerve pathways up to the brainstem.

52. **Auditory Processing Disorder (APD)** - A condition where the brain has difficulty processing auditory information.

53. **Auditory Prosthesis** - Any device that aids hearing, including cochlear implants and bone anchored hearing aids.

54. **Aural Fullness** - A feeling of pressure in the ears that may occur with changes in hearing or vestibular disorders.

55. **Binaural Hearing** - The ability to use both ears to hear, which helps in sound localization and understanding speech in noise.

56. **Caloric Test** - A test that uses changes in temperature to assess the response of the vestibular system.

57. **Deafness** - A significant hearing impairment that may prevent speech communication; can be partial or total.

58. **Ear Flap** - The outer part of the ear that helps to collect sound waves; another term for the pinna.

59. **Ear Trumpet** - A historical device used to assist hearing by collecting sound waves and directing them into the ear canal.

60. **Echoic Memory** - A component of sensory memory that holds auditory information.

61. **Endaural Phenomena** - Sounds perceived from within the ear itself, such as those caused by internal functions or disorders.

62. **Engelmann's Bone** - A term sometimes used to describe the stapes bone due to its critical role in hearing.

63. **Entrainment** - The synchronization of neuronal activity to an external auditory rhythm.

64. **Eustachian Tube Dysfunction** - A condition where the Eustachian tube does not open and close properly, affecting ear pressure and hearing.

65. **Evoked Auditory Potentials** - Electrical potentials recorded from the auditory cortex in response to sound stimulation.

66. **Frequency Discrimination** - The ability to distinguish different frequencies of sound waves.

67. **Gain Control** - In hearing aids, a feature that adjusts the volume of sound automatically based on the level of background noise.

68. **Hearing Conservation** - Programs and strategies aimed at preventing hearing loss due to noise exposure.

69. **Hearing Threshold** - The smallest level of sound that an individual can hear.

70. **Hereditary Hearing Impairment** - Hearing loss that occurs due to genetic factors or conditions inherited from parents.

71. **High-Frequency Hearing Loss** - A hearing impairment where it is difficult to hear sounds in the higher frequency range.

72. **Implantable Hearing Devices** - Devices that are surgically placed to improve hearing, unlike traditional hearing aids that are worn externally.

73. **Infrasound** - Sound waves with frequencies below the lower limit of human audibility.

74. **Interaural Time Difference (ITD)** - The difference in time for a sound to reach each ear, used to localize sound sources.

75. **Kernicterus** - A form of brain damage caused by excessive jaundice, which can lead to auditory nerve damage.

76. **Loudness Recruitment** - A phenomenon where the perceived loudness of sound increases faster than normal.

77. **Masking** - The process by which the perception of one sound is affected by the presence of another sound.

78. **Mastoid Process** - A portion of the temporal bone of the skull located behind the ear, which contains air spaces that communicate with the middle ear.

79. **Noise-Induced Hearing Loss (NIHL)** - Hearing loss caused by exposure to harmful sounds.

80. **Occlusion Effect** - An increase in the perception of low-frequency sounds when the ear canal is blocked.

81. **Otalgia** - Ear pain or earache.

82. **Otoendoscopy** - The use of an endoscope for visual examination of the ear's interior, especially the middle and inner ear.

83. **Otoplasty** - Surgical alteration of the external ear, often performed for cosmetic reasons or to correct deformities.

84. **Ototoxicity** - Ear poisoning which occurs when the inner ear is damaged by substances like certain medications.

85. **Perforated Eardrum** - A tear or hole in the eardrum, which can affect hearing and make the middle ear vulnerable to infections.

86. **Phase Locking** - The ability of auditory nerve fibers to fire at a particular point in the sound wave cycle, crucial for processing sound frequencies.

87. **Pitch Perception** - The ability to perceive how high or low a sound is.

88. **Pure Tone Audiometry** - A hearing test that uses pure tone sounds to find the quietest sound that a person can hear at various frequencies.

89. **Real Ear Measurement** - The measurement of sound levels in the ear canal when a hearing aid is worn, used to ensure the hearing aid is properly adjusted.

90. **Reflex Decay** - A decrease in the strength of the acoustic reflex over time when a continuous sound is presented.

91. **Retrocochlear Hearing Loss** - Hearing loss caused by damage to the neural pathways beyond the cochlea, including the auditory nerve and brain.

92. **Round Window** - A membrane-covered opening in the bone of the middle ear that responds to fluid vibrations in the cochlea.

93. **Semicircular Canals** - Three fluid-filled loops in the inner ear that are responsible for maintaining balance.

94. **Sound Localization** - The process by which the position of a sound source is determined.

95. **Speech Audiometry** - A method used to measure how well a person can understand speech and at what levels.

96. **Speech Discrimination** - The ability to distinguish between different sounds or words.

97. **Stapedius Muscle** - A small muscle in the ear that helps to dampen the vibrations of the stapes bone, protecting the inner ear from loud noises.

98. **Tectorial Membrane** - A structure in the cochlea that contacts hair cells, playing a crucial role in the sensory transduction of sound.

99. **Temporal Bone** - The bone of the skull where the inner ear is located.

100.   **Threshold Shift** - A temporary or permanent change in the threshold of hearing sensitivity.

101.   **Timbre** - The quality of a sound that distinguishes different types of sound production, such as voices or musical instruments.

102.   **Tone Decay Test** - A test to assess the ability of the auditory system to sustain a response to a continuous sound.

103.   **Tragus** - A small pointed eminence of the external ear, located in front of the ear canal.

104.   **Transverse Temporal Gyrus** - An area of the brain where primary auditory processing occurs.

105.   **Tympanic Cavity** - The small air-filled chamber of the middle ear that houses the ossicles.

106.   **Utricle** - One of the two otolithic organs located in the vestibule of the inner ear, used to sense gravity and linear acceleration.

107.   **Vestibular Evoked Myogenic Potential (VEMP)** - A test that measures the reflexive responses of muscles in the neck and eyes to sounds, used to assess the vestibular system.

108.   **Vestibular Neuritis** - Inflammation of the vestibular nerve, typically causing vertigo.

109.   **Vestibular Rehabilitation** - Therapy aimed at alleviating the symptoms of vestibular disorders through specific exercises.

110.   **Volume Acuity** - The ability to perceive changes in the loudness of sounds.

111.   **Wax Blockage** - Accumulation of earwax that can block the ear canal and impair hearing.

112.   **Weber Test** - A quick screening test for hearing that can detect unilateral (one-sided) conductive hearing loss and sensorineural hearing loss.

113.   **Zygomatic Bone** - A bone that forms the prominence of the cheek; involved in the attachment of muscles associated with the outer ear.

114.   **Auditory Fatigue** - Temporary hearing loss caused by prolonged exposure to high-intensity sounds.

115.   **Bezold-Brücke Phenomenon** - A phenomenon where the perceived hue of colors changes as brightness changes, similar to how pitch perception can change with loudness.

Olfactory and Gustatory Systems

1. **Olfactory Bulb** - A brain structure responsible for receiving neural input about odours detected by cells in the nasal cavity.

2. **Olfactory Epithelium** - A specialized epithelial tissue inside the nasal cavity that is involved in smell.

3. **Olfactory Receptors** - Proteins in the cell membranes of olfactory neurons sensitive to chemical compounds.

4. **Olfactory Nerve (Cranial Nerve I)** - The nerve that carries smell information from the olfactory receptors to the brain.

5. **Anosmia** - Inability or loss of the sense of smell.

6. **Hyposmia** - Reduced ability to smell.

7. **Dysosmia** - When things smell differently than they should (distorted sense of smell).

8. **Phantosmia** - "Smelling" odors that aren't actually present (olfactory hallucination).

9. **Olfactory Cortex** - Part of the cerebral cortex involved in processing smell.

10. **Nasal Cavity** - The large air-filled space above and behind the nose in the middle of the face.

11. **Gustatory Cells** - Sensory cells within the taste buds that are responsible for the sensation of taste.

12. **Taste Buds** - Sensory organs on the tongue and other parts of the mouth that are involved in tasting.

13. **Papillae** - Small bumps on the tongue that contain taste buds.

14. **Fungiform Papillae** - Mushroom-shaped structures on the upper surface of the tongue that house taste buds.

15. **Foliate Papillae** - Folds on the sides of the tongue that contain taste buds.

16. **Circumvallate Papillae** - Large circular structures on the back of the tongue that contain taste buds.

17. **Gustatory Pathway** - The neural pathway that transmits taste information from the tongue to the brain.

18. **Taste Pore** - An opening on the surface of the taste bud through which gustatory hairs project.

19. **Gustatory Hairs** - Microscopic hairs that protrude from gustatory cells into the taste pores and are stimulated by food chemicals.

20. **Gustatory Cortex** - Area of the brain that processes taste information.

21. **Ageusia** - Loss of taste functions of the tongue, particularly the inability to detect sweetness, sourness, bitterness, saltiness, and umami.

22. **Hypogeusia** - Reduced ability to taste things.

23. **Dysgeusia** - Distorted sense of taste.

24. **Chemosensory System** - The sensory system that combines the senses of smell and taste.

25. **Olfactory Tract** - A bilateral structure that carries information from the olfactory bulb to other parts of the brain.

26. **Gustatory Nerve** - Nerves that carry taste sensations to the brain (part of facial, glossopharyngeal, and vagus nerves).

27. **Flavor** - The combined sense of taste, smell, and other sensations (such as texture and temperature) that is crucial to experiencing food.

28. **Umami** - One of the five basic tastes, recognizing the flavor of glutamates, commonly found in meat and some artificial flavorings.

29. **Nasal Conchae** - Long, narrow shelves in the nasal cavity that increase its surface area.

30. **Superior, Middle, and Inferior Nasal Conchae** - Structures that regulate air flow through the nasal passages and increase epithelial area for smelling.

31. **Cribriform Plate** - Part of the ethmoid bone of the skull, where the olfactory nerves pass from the nasal cavity to the olfactory bulb.

32. **Neural Adaptation** - The phenomenon whereby sensory receptors become less sensitive to constant stimuli.

33. **Sensory Integration** - The process by which the brain combines information from different sensory systems.

34. **Primary Olfactory Cortex** - The first region within the cerebral cortex which receives olfactory information from the olfactory bulb.

35. **Olfactory Gland (Bowman's Gland)** - Secretes mucus that helps dissolve odor molecules so that they can bind to olfactory receptors.

36. **Taste Transduction** - The process by which a taste stimulus is converted into an electrical signal in the gustatory system.

37. **Saliva** - Fluid in the mouth that helps dissolve food chemicals to be tasted.

38. **Orthonasal Olfaction** - Detection of an odor through sniffing in through the nostrils.

39. **Retronasal Olfaction** - Detection of an odorant when it is released fromfood in the mouth during chewing and swallowing, allowing for the perception of flavor through the back of the oral cavity.

40. **Taste Modality** - Classification of taste perception, typically as sweet, sour, bitter, salty, and umami.

41. **Gustducin** - A protein involved in the signal transduction pathways for taste.

42. **Lingual Nerve** - A branch of the mandibular nerve (cranial nerve V3) that carries taste fibers from the front two-thirds of the tongue.

43. **Chorda Tympani** - A branch of the facial nerve (cranial nerve VII) that carries taste sensations from the anterior two-thirds of the tongue.

44. **Glossopharyngeal Nerve (Cranial Nerve IX)** - Carries taste sensations from the posterior one-third of the tongue.

45. **Vagus Nerve (Cranial Nerve X)** - Carries taste sensations from the back of the mouth and throat.

46. **Insular Cortex** - Part of the cerebral cortex involved in the perception and integrated experience of taste, smell, and visceral sensations.

47. **Solitary Tract** - A structure in the brainstem that receives incoming taste sensation.

48. **Solitary Nucleus** - The nucleus within the solitary tract where taste and visceral sensory information is processed.

49. **Flavor Profile** - The combined array of taste, smell, and other sensory characteristics of a particular food or drink.

50. **Cephalic Phase Responses** - Physiological responses to the sight, smell, or thought of food, preparing the body for digestion.

51. **Neurogastronomy** - The study of how the brain perceives flavor.

52. **Palate** - The roof of the mouth, separating the oral cavity from the nasal cavity, involved in taste and tactile sensations.

53. **Olfactory Projection Pathways** - Routes along which olfactory information is sent from the olfactory bulb to higher regions of the brain.

54. **Taste Threshold** - The minimum concentration of a substance required to produce a perceptible taste.

55. **Salty Taste** - One of the basic tastes; primarily produced by the presence of sodium ions.

56. **Sweet Taste** - Taste sensation produced by sugars and substances that mimic the properties of sugars.

57. **Bitter Taste** - Basic taste modality associated with many compounds, often considered unpleasant, and is thought to be a protective function against ingestion of toxins.

58. **Sour Taste** - Taste modality that detects acidity; the taste sensation produced by hydrogen ions.

59. **Olfactometer** - An instrument used to detect and measure odor dilution.

60. **Gustatory System Disorders** - Conditions affecting the sense of taste, including genetic and acquired disorders.

61. **Taste Bud Regeneration** - The process by which taste cells are regularly replaced, which occurs approximately every 10 days.

62. **Anatomical Taste Map** - The outdated concept that different regions of the tongue are responsible for perceiving different tastes.

63. **Olfactory Memory** - The storage and recall of the smells experienced; closely linked to emotional memory.

64. **Ethmoid Sinus** - One of the paranasal sinuses, its inflammation can affect the sense of smell due to its proximity to the olfactory bulb.

65. **Mucous Membrane** - The membrane lining the nose and mouth, which secretes mucus that helps moisten and protect the surface.

66. **Olfactory Discrimination** - The ability to distinguish between and identify different odors.

67. **Taste Intensity** - The strength of a taste sensation, which can be influenced by temperature, texture, and other factors.

68. **Olfactory Saturation** - A temporary, adaptive reduction in sensitivity to an odor after prolonged exposure.

69. **Gustatory Acuity** - The ability to detect and recognize differing levels of taste intensities and qualities.

70. **Nasal Septum** - The bone and cartilage wall that divides the nasal cavity into two nostrils, crucial for proper airflow and nasal function.

71. **Olfactory Assays** - Laboratory methods used to measure and analyze the sense of smell.

72. **Taste Adaptation** - The phenomenon where the perception of a taste decreases when the stimulus is continuously present.

73. **Vomeronasal Organ (Jacobson's Organ)** - A part of the olfactory system in many animals (largely non-functional in humans) used to detect pheromones.

74. **Pheromones** - Chemicals capable of acting like hormones outside the body, influencing the behavior of other individuals.

75. **Chemoreception** - The physiological response to chemical stimuli, which includes the senses of taste and smell.

76. **Olfactory Conditioning** - The process by which behaviors are modified using odors as the conditioned stimuli.

77. **Tonsils** - Lymphatic tissue located at the back of the throat which can influence taste if swollen or infected.

78. **Palatine Tonsil** - Located on the sides of the throat, these can influence taste sensations if inflamed.

79. **Nasopharynx** - The upper part of the pharynx, connecting the nasal cavity above the soft palate.

80. **Soft Palate** - The soft tissue constituting the back of the roof of the mouth.

81. **Hard Palate** - The bony front part of the palate.

82. **Nasal Polyps** - Noncancerous growths on the lining of the nasal passages or sinuses, which can affect smell and taste by blocking nasal passages.

83. **Sinusitis** - Inflammation of the sinuses, often causing a temporary loss of smell and altered taste.

84. **Adenoids** - A mass of lymphoid tissue located at the back of the nasal cavity; inflammation can affect breathing and the sense of smell.

85. **Turbinates** - Long, narrow bones that protrude into the nasal cavity; they increase the surface area of the nose and help warm and moisten the air.

86. **Taste-Smell Confusion** - When the senses of taste and smell are confused; common in neurological disorders.

87. **Pharynx** - The membrane-lined cavity behind the nose and mouth, connecting them to the esophagus.

88. **Lacrimal Glands** - Glands located in the upper outer region of the orbit of the eye that produce tears, which can influence the nasal cavity through the nasolacrimal duct.

89. **Taste-Smell Synthesis** - The blending of taste and smell perceptions into a single flavor perception.

90. **Olfactory Hallucination** - The perception of smells that aren't present, often occurring in medical conditions like epilepsy or migraines.

91. **Gustation** - The technical term for the sense of taste.

92. **Olfaction** - The technical term for the sense of smell.

93. **Intermodal Sensory Integration** - The process by which the brain integrates information from different sensory modalities, such as taste and smell.

94. **Tactile Sensations in Taste** - The role of touch or texture in the perception of food and its flavor.

95. **Thermal Sensations in Taste** - The impact of temperature on taste perception (e.g., cold ice cream vs. hot coffee).

96. **Olfactory Fatigue** - The temporary, normal inability to distinguish a particular odor after a prolonged exposure to that airborne compound.

97. **Nasal Mucosa** - The mucous membrane lining the nasal cavity, involved in the sense of smell and in filtering the air breathed.

98. **Olfactory Ensheathing Cells** - Specialized cells that help olfactory nerve fibers in the nasal cavity to enter the brain; they have potential use in regenerative medicine.

99. **Olfactory Marker Protein** - A protein found in olfactory neurons, useful in olfactory research.

100. **Sour Receptors** - Specific receptors on taste cells that detect acidic compounds.

101. **Salt Receptors** - Taste receptors that detect the presence of sodium and other ions.

102. **Bitter Receptors** - Receptors on taste cells that identify potentially harmful toxins.

103. **Sweet Receptors** - Receptors that identify sugars and substances that have a similar structure to sugars.

104. **Umami Receptors** - Receptors that detect amino acids, typically associated with the flavor enhancer monosodium glutamate.

105. **Gustatory Hair Cells** - Cells in taste buds that respond to chemical stimuli and are involved in the process of taste perception.

106. **Olfactory Microvilli** - Tiny hair-like structures in the olfactory system that increase the surface area for detecting odors.

107. **Taste Impairment** - Any disturbance or partial loss of the ability to taste.

108. **Olfactory Impairment** - Any reduction in the ability to smell.

109. **Olfactory Cortex Mapping** - The process of identifying and detailing the specific regions of the brain associated with the perception of smells.

110. **Neurogastronomy** - The interdisciplinary study that explores how the brain creates the perception of flavor.

111. **Flavor Profile Analysis** - The technique of breaking down and describing the specific flavors in food or drink.

112. **Aroma Compounds** - Chemicals that are responsible for the odors and flavors in foods and beverages.

113. **Volatile Organic Compounds (VOCs)** - Organic chemicals that have a high vapor pressure at room temperature, critical in the perception of aroma.

114. **Retronasal Olfaction** - The process of smelling through the mouth while eating, which contributes to the perception of flavor.

115. **Ortho-Nasal Olfaction** - The process of smelling through the nose, which is the traditional way of perceiving smells.

Musculoskeletal System Terminology

1. **Osteology** - The study of bones.

2. **Myology** - The study of muscles.

3. **Arthrology** - The study of joints.

4. **Ligament** - Connective tissue that connects bones at a joint.

5. **Tendon** - Connective tissue that attaches muscle to bone.

6. **Cartilage** - A smooth elastic tissue that covers and protects the ends of bones at joints.

7. **Synovial Fluid** - Lubricating fluid within a joint.

8. **Bursa** - A fluid-filled sac that reduces friction between tissues of the body.

9. **Axial Skeleton** - The part of the skeleton that consists of the bones of the head and trunk.

10. **Appendicular Skeleton** - The part of the skeleton that includes the bones of the limbs.

11. **Bone Marrow** - The soft tissue inside bones where blood cells are produced.

12. **Compact Bone** - Dense bone tissue that forms the outer layer of a bone.

13. **Spongy Bone** - Porous bone tissue that is found inside bones.

14. **Osteocyte** - A mature bone cell.

15. **Osteoblast** - A cell that produces new bone tissue.

16. **Osteoclast** - A cell that breaks down bone tissue.

17. **Osteoporosis** - A condition in which bones become weak and brittle.

18. **Fracture** - A break in a bone.

19. **Dislocation** - Displacement of a bone from its joint.

20. **Sprain** - Stretching or tearing of ligaments.

21. **Strain** - Stretching or tearing of muscles or tendons.

22. **Osteoarthritis** - Degenerative joint disease.

23. **Rheumatoid Arthritis** - An autoimmune disorder that primarily affects joints.

24. **Scoliosis** - A lateral curvature of the spine.

25. **Kyphosis** - Excessive outward curvature of the spine, causing hunching.

26. **Lordosis** - Excessive inward curvature of the spine.

27. **Intervertebral Disc** - A disc that acts as a shock absorber between the bones in the spine.

28. **Nucleus Pulposus** - The jelly-like center of an intervertebral disc.

29. **Annulus Fibrosus** - The tough outer layer of an intervertebral disc.

30. **Vertebra** - An individual bone in the spine.

31. **Cervical Vertebrae** - The vertebrae of the neck.

32. **Thoracic Vertebrae** - The vertebrae of the upper back.

33. **Lumbar Vertebrae** - The vertebrae of the lower back.

34. **Sacrum** - A bone formed from fused vertebrae below the lumbar spine.

35. **Coccyx** - The tailbone, formed from fused vertebrae at the base of the spine.

36. **Scapula** - Shoulder blade.

37. **Clavicle** - Collarbone.

38. **Humerus** - Upper arm bone.

39. **Radius** - One of the forearm bones, on the thumb side.

40. **Ulna** - One of the forearm bones, on the little finger side.

41. **Carpals** - Wrist bones.

42. **Metacarpals** - Bones of the hand.

43. **Phalanges** - Finger and toe bones.

44. **Femur** - Thigh bone.

45. **Patella** - Kneecap.

46. **Tibia** - Shin bone.

47. **Fibula** - Calf bone.

48. **Tarsals** - Ankle bones.

49. **Metatarsals** - Foot bones.

50. **Glenoid Cavity** - The socket in the scapula for the head of the humerus.

51. **Acetabulum** - The hip socket.

52. **Synovial Joint** - A freely movable joint.

53. **Fibrous Joint** - A joint connected by fibrous connective tissue.

54. **Cartilaginous Joint** - A joint where the bones are joined by cartilage.

55. **Ball and Socket Joint** - A joint in which a ball-shaped surface of one bone fits into a cup-like depression of another bone.

56. **Hinge Joint** - A joint that allows movement in one direction.

57. **Pivot Joint** - A joint that allows rotational movement.

58. **Saddle Joint** - A joint that allows movements in two directions.

59. **Condyloid Joint** - A joint that allows movement but no rotation.
    60.61. **Ellipsoid Joint** - A type of synovial joint that allows all types of movement except axial rotation.

60. **Plane Joint** - A type of joint that allows only gliding movements.

61. **Spinal Foramen** - The hole in the center of the vertebra through which the spinal cord passes.

62. **Foramen Magnum** - A large opening in the base of the skull through which the brain connects to the spinal cord.

63. **Fascia** - A band or sheet of connective tissue, primarily collagen, beneath the skin that attaches, stabilizes, encloses, and separates muscles and other internal organs.

64. **Muscle Fiber** - A single muscle cell, known for its elongated shape.

65. **Myofibril** - Any of the elongated contractile threads found in striated muscle cells.

66. **Sarcomere** - The basic unit of a muscle's cross-striated myofibril.

67. **Actin** - A protein that forms (together with myosin) the contractile filaments of muscle cells.

68. **Myosin** - A fibrous protein that forms (with actin) the contractile filaments of muscle cells and is also involved in motion in other types of cells.

69. **Trophic** - Relating to feeding and nutrition; often used in context to describe factors affecting the growth and maintenance of tissues.

70. **Atrophy** - The reduction in size or wasting away of an organ or tissue from a lack of use or nutritional support.

71. **Hypertrophy** - The enlargement of an organ or tissue from the increase in size of its cells.

72. **Rhabdomyolysis** - A condition in which damaged skeletal muscle breaks down rapidly.

73. **Myalgia** - Muscle pain.

74. **Osteomalacia** - Softening of the bones, typically through a deficiency of vitamin D or calcium.

75. **Osteogenesis Imperfecta** - A genetic disorder characterized by bones that break easily, often with little or no apparent cause.

76. **Osteomyelitis** - Inflammation of bone or bone marrow, usually due to infection.

77. **Chondrocyte** - A cell that has secreted the matrix of cartilage and become embedded in it.

78. **Periosteum** - A dense layer of vascular connective tissue enveloping the bones except at the surfaces of the joints.

79. **Endosteum** - A thin vascular membrane of connective tissue that lines the inner surface of the bony tissue that forms the medullary cavity of long bones.

80. **Epiphysis** - The end part of a long bone, initially growing separately from the shaft.

81. **Diaphysis** - The shaft or central part of a long bone.

82. **Epiphyseal Plate** - Also known as the growth plate, it is a hyaline cartilage plate in the metaphysis at each end of a long bone.

83. **Metaphysis** - The narrow portion of a long bone between the epiphysis and the diaphysis.

84. **Aponeurosis** - A type of fibrous tissue that takes the place of a tendon in sheet-like muscles having a wide area of attachment.

85. **Synarthrosis** - A type of joint which permits very little or no movement under normal conditions, most are fibrous joints.

86. **Amphiarthrosis** - A type of joint that allows only slight movement.

87. **Myositis** - Inflammation or degeneration of muscle tissue.

88. **Sarcopenia** - The loss of muscle mass and strength that occurs with aging.

89. **Dystrophy** - A disorder in which an organ or tissue of the body wastes away.

90. **Gout** - A form of arthritis characterized by severe pain, redness, and tenderness in joints, caused by crystals that form in and around the joint.

91. **Bone Density** - A measure of bone strength, the amount of mineral matter per square centimeter of bones.

92. **Bone Scan** - A nuclear scanning test that identifies new areas of bone growth or breakdown.

93. **Rickets** - A disease of children caused by vitamin D deficiency, characterized by imperfect calcification, softening, and distortion of the bones typically resulting in bow legs.

94. **Leukemia** - A type of cancer that affects the blood and bone marrow.

95. **Muscular Dystrophy** - A group of genetic diseases that cause progressive weakness and loss of muscle mass.

96. **Myopathy** - Any disease of the muscle.

97. **Orthopedic** - Pertaining to the correction of deformities of bones or muscles.

98. **Rheumatology** - The study and treatment of rheumatic diseases and musculoskeletal disorders.

99. **Prosthesis** - An artificial device to replace a missing part of the body.

100. **Osteotomy** - A surgical operation whereby a bone is cut to shorten, lengthen, or change its alignment.

101. **Arthroscopy** - A surgical procedure for diagnosing and treating joint problems.

102. **Laminectomy** - A surgical operation to remove the back part of the vertebra that covers your spinal canal.

103.   **Fusion (Spinal Fusion)** - Surgical procedure to connect two or more vertebrae in the spine, eliminating motion between them.

104.   **Bone Graft** - Surgical procedure using transplanted bone to repair and rebuild diseased or damaged bones.

105.   **Chondromalacia** - Softening of the cartilage under the kneecap.

106.   **Meniscus** - A crescent-shaped cartilage found in the knee.

107.   **Rotator Cuff** - A group of muscles and their tendons that act to stabilize the shoulder.

108.   **Plantar Fasciitis** - Inflammation of a thick band of tissue that connects the heel bone to the toes.

109.   **Achilles Tendonitis** - Inflammation of the Achilles tendon, typically caused by overuse.

110.   **Hallux Valgus** - A bunion, or a misalignment of the big toe joint.

111.   **Carpal Tunnel Syndrome** - A condition caused by compression of the median nerve in the carpal tunnel and characterized by numbness, tingling, and pain in the hand.

112.   **Shin Splints** - Pain along the inner edge of the shinbone (tibia).

113.   **Lateral Epicondylitis** - Commonly known as tennis elbow, a condition involving the outer elbow tendons.

114.   **Medial Epicondylitis** - Known as golfer's elbow, affects tendons on the inner side of the elbow.

115.   **Ankylosing Spondylitis** - A type of arthritis that causes chronic inflammation of the spine and the sacroiliac joints.

Integumentary System Terminology

1. **Epidermis** - The outermost layer of skin.

2. **Dermis** - The layer of skin beneath the epidermis that contains hair follicles and glands.

3. **Hypodermis** - The deeper subcutaneous tissue made of fat and connective tissue.

4. **Keratin** - A protein that protects epithelial cells from damage or stress.

5. **Melanin** - A pigment that gives the skin, hair, and eyes their color.

6. **Sebaceous Glands** - Oil-producing glands in the skin.

7. **Sweat Glands** - Glands that release sweat to help regulate body temperature.

8. **Hair Follicle** - The sac within the skin from which hair grows.

9. **Nail Bed** - The skin beneath the nail plate.

10. **Cuticle** - The layer of clear skin located along the bottom edge of your finger or toe nails.

11. **Dermatology** - The branch of medicine dealing with the skin and its diseases.

12. **Acne** - A skin condition characterized by red pimples, often due to inflamed or infected sebaceous glands.

13. **Eczema** - A condition that causes inflamed, itchy, cracked, and rough skin.

14. **Psoriasis** - A skin disease marked by red, itchy, scaly patches.

15. **Dermatitis** - Inflammation of the skin.

16. **Melanoma** - A type of skin cancer developing from the pigment-containing cells known as melanocytes.

17. **Basal Cell Carcinoma** - A form of skin cancer that begins in the basal cells.

18. **Squamous Cell Carcinoma** - A form of skin cancer that begins in the squamous cells.

19. **Lipoma** - A benign tumor made of fat tissue.

20. **Mole (Nevus)** - A small, often dark brown, spot on the skin formed from clusters of pigmented cells.

21. **Wart** - A small, hard, benign growth on the skin, caused by a virus.

22. **Papule** - A small, raised bump on the skin that is usually less than 1 centimeter around.

23. **Macule** - A flat, distinct, colored area of skin that is usually less than 10 millimeters wide.

24. **Patch** - A large macule.

25. **Nodule** - A larger, firm lesion that is deeper than a papule.

26. **Wheal** - A raised, itchy area of skin that is often a sign of an allergic reaction.

27. **Ulcer** - A deep loss of skin surface that may extend to the dermis and frequently bleeds and scars.

28. **Scar** - A mark left on the skin or within body tissue where a wound, burn, or sore has not healed completely and fibrous connective tissue has developed.

29. **Keloid** - A raised scar after an injury has healed.

30. **Fissure** - A small tear in the skin.

31. **Abscess** - A collection of pus that has built up within the tissue of the body.

32. **Cyst** - A sac-like pocket of membranous tissue containing fluid, air, or other substances.

33. **Petechiae** - Small red or purple spots caused by bleeding into the skin.

34. **Purpura** - Larger purple areas of bleeding into the skin.

35. **Ecchymosis** - A large bruise.

36. **Tinea** - A fungal infection of the skin; also known as ringworm.

37. **Albinism** - A group of inherited disorders characterized by little or no melanin production.

38. **Vitiligo** - A condition in which the skin loses its pigment cells (melanocytes).

39. **Hirsutism** - Excessive hair growth on women in those parts of the body where hair is normally absent or minimal.

40. **Alopecia** - Hair loss from the scalp or elsewhere on the body.

41. **Comedo** - A clogged hair follicle (pore) in the skin, seen in acne; can be open (blackhead) or closed (whitehead).

42. **Stratum Corneum** - The outermost layer of the epidermis, consisting of dead cells (corneocytes).

43. **Stratum Basale** - The deepest layer of the epidermis where new skin cells are generated.

44. **Hyperkeratosis** - Thickening of the outer layer of the skin, often associated with the presence of an abnormal quantity of keratin.

45. **Hyperpigmentation** - Darkening of an area of skin caused by increased melanin.

46. **Hypopigmentation** - Lightening of skin, caused by reduced melanin production.

47. **Sunburn** - Redness and irritation of the skin caused by excessive exposure to ultraviolet (UV) rays.

48. **Dermal Papillae** - Small, nipple-like extensions of the dermis into the epidermis.

49. **Melanocyte** - A cell in the basal layer that produces melanin.

50. **Keratinocyte** - The primary type of cell found in the epidermis, responsible for forming the barrier against environmental damage.

51. **Langerhans Cell** - A type of dendritic cell (immune cell) found in the skin, playing an important role in the immune response.

52. **Merkel Cell** - A type of skin cell associated with touch sensation.

53. **Seborrheic Keratosis** - A common noncancerous skin growth in older adults.

54. **Skin Tag** - A small, benign tumor that forms primarily in areas where the skin forms creases or rubs together.

55. **Xerosis** - The medical term for dry skin.

56. **Pruritus** - Itchy skin.

57. **Urticaria** - Also known as hives, a skin rash triggered by a reaction to food, medicine, or other irritants.

58. **Rosacea** - A chronic skin condition that causes redness and visible blood vessels in your face.

59. **Impetigo** - A highly contagious skin infection that causes red sores on the face.

60. **Cellulitis** - A common bacterial skin infection.

61. **Herpes Zoster** - Also known as shingles, a viral infection that causes a painful rash.

62. **Varicella** - Chickenpox, a viral infection causing a mild fever and a rash of itchy inflamed pimples.

63. **Pressure Ulcer** - Injury to skin and underlying tissue resulting from prolonged pressure on the skin.

64. **Decubitus Ulcer** - Another term for pressure ulcer, often used in medical contexts.

65. **Skin Biopsy** - A diagnostic test involving the removal of cells or skin samples for examination.

66. **Dermabrasion** - A procedure to diminish the appearance of imperfections, such as scars or wrinkles on the skin.

67. **Mohs Surgery** - A precise surgical technique used to treat skin cancer.

68. **Botox** - Injections used cosmetically to remove wrinkles by temporarily paralyzing facial muscles.

69. **Fillers** - Substances injected into the skin to fill wrinkles and add volume.

70. **Laser Resurfacing** - A treatment to reduce facial wrinkles and skin irregularities by using concentrated light.

71. **Cryotherapy** - Treatment using extreme cold, often with liquid nitrogen, to treat skin conditions.

72. **Phototherapy** - Treatment using ultraviolet light, often for conditions like psoriasis.

73. **Electrodesiccation** - A procedure that uses electric current to remove specific skin lesions.

74. **Skin Flap Surgery** - A surgical procedure where skin and its underlying structures are moved to cover a defect.

75. **Skin Graft** - Transplanting skin from one area of the body to another to replace damaged or missing skin.

76. **Dermatographism** - A condition also known as skin writing, where slight scratches turn into a raised red reaction.

77. **Angioedema** - Swelling in the deep layers of the skin, often seen with hives.

78. **Keratosis Pilaris** - A condition that causes rough patches and small, acne-like bumps on the skin.

79. **Actinic Keratosis** - A rough, scaly patch on the skin that develops from years of sun exposure.

80. **Onychomycosis** - Fungal infection of the nails.

81. **Paronychia** - An infection of the skin around the nail.

82. **Dermatofibroma** - A common benign skin nodule seen on the legs.

83. **Epidermolysis Bullosa** - A group of genetic conditions that cause the skin to be very fragile and to blister easily.

84. **Ichthyosis** - A family of genetic skin disorders characterized by dry, scaling skin.

85. **Lichen Planus** - A condition that causes swelling and irritation in the skin, hair, nails, and mucous membranes.

86. **Pityriasis Rosea** - A rash that usually begins as a large circular or oval spot on your chest, abdomen or back.

87. **Scabies** - An infestation of the skin by the human itch mite.

88. **Sclerotherapy** - A procedure used to treat blood vessel malformations (vascular malformations) and also used in the treatment of varicose veins.

89. **Spider Veins** - Small, dilated blood vessels near the surface of the skin.

90. **Varicose Veins** - Large, swollen blood vessels that typically appear in the legs and feet.

91. **Hyperhidrosis** - Excessive sweating.

92. **Anhidrosis** - Absence of sweating.

93. **Dyschromias** - Disorders of pigmentation in the skin.

94. **Freckles (Ephelides)** - Small brown spots on the skin, often highly visible and commonly appearing on people with a fair complexion.

95. **Lentigines** - Small pigmented spots on the skin with a clearly defined edge, surrounded by normal-appearing skin.

96. **Nevus of Ota** - A bluish pigmentation that appears on the face, most often affecting people of Asian descent.

97. **Port-wine Stain** - A birthmark in which swollen blood vessels create a reddish-purplish discoloration of the skin.

98. **Hemangioma** - A benign tumor of blood vessels, often appearing as a red birthmark.

99. **Dermatosis Papulosa Nigra** - Small, black marks typically found on the cheeks of people with darker skin.

100. **Xanthelasma** - Yellowish plaques on eyelids or around eyes, commonly associated with lipid disorders.

101. **Seborrheic Dermatitis** - A chronic form of eczema that appears on the body parts where there are a lot of oil-producing (sebaceous) glands like the upper back, nose and scalp.

102. **Acrochordons** - Small, benign growths that typically appear in areas where the skin forms creases, commonly known as skin tags.

103. **Candidiasis** - Fungal infection caused by yeasts from the genus Candida, commonly affecting the skin.

104. **Dermatophytosis** - Fungal infection of the skin, hair, or nails commonly referred to as ringworm.

105. **Intertrigo** - A rash (dermatitis) that appears in the body folds.

106. **Kaposi's Sarcoma** - A type of cancer that forms in the lining of blood and lymph vessels; often appears as purple patches on the skin or mucous membranes.

107. **Liposuction** - A cosmetic procedure used to remove unwanted body fat.

108. **Necrotizing Fasciitis** - A serious bacterial infection that destroys tissue under the skin.

109. **Pilonidal Cyst** - A chronic skin infection at the crease of the buttocks near the coccyx (tailbone).

110. **Plantar Warts** - Hard, grainy growths that appear on the heels or balls of the feet.

111. **Psoralen Plus Ultraviolet A (PUVA)** - A form of treatment using a photosensitizing drug and exposure to ultraviolet A light.

112. **Reticulate** - A network-like pattern, often used to describe certain patterns of skin lesion.

113. **RhinoPhyma** - A form of rosacea characterized by an enlarged, bulbous, and red nose.

114. **Solar Lentigines** - Often called 'liver spots' or 'age spots,' these are related to sun exposure.

115. **Striae** - Also known as stretch marks, these are streaks or lines that appear on the skin, usually as a result of rapid stretching.

Reproductive System

1. **Gonads** - Organs that produce gametes; testes in males and ovaries in females.

2. **Gametes** - Reproductive cells (sperm in males and ova in females).

3. **Fertilization** - The union of a sperm and an ovum to form a zygote.

4. **Zygote** - The cell resulting from the fusion of an ovum and a sperm.

5. **Embryo** - The developing organism from fertilization until about eight weeks.

6. **Fetus** - The developing organism from the end of the eighth week until birth.

7. **Uterus** - The female organ where the embryo and fetus develop until birth.

8. **Endometrium** - The lining of the uterus, which thickens during the menstrual cycle.

9. **Menstruation** - The shedding of the uterine lining out of the vagina.

10. **Ovulation** - The release of an ovum from one of the ovaries.

11. **Fallopian Tubes** - Tubes that carry ova from the ovaries to the uterus.

12. **Cervix** - The lower, narrow part of the uterus that opens into the vagina.

13. **Vagina** - The canal leading from the cervix to the outside of the body.

14. **Menarche** - The first menstrual period in a female.

15. **Menopause** - The end of menstruation and reproductive capacity in a female.

16. **Testes** - The male reproductive organs that produce sperm and testosterone.

17. **Spermatozoa** - The male reproductive cells commonly known as sperm.

18. **Epididymis** - A duct behind the testes, where sperm mature and are stored.

19. **Vas Deferens** - The duct that conveys sperm from the testicle to the urethra.

20. **Seminal Vesicles** - Glands that secrete fluid that partly composes semen.

21. **Prostate Gland** - A gland in males that contributes to the seminal fluid.

22. **Urethra** - The duct through which urine is conveyed out of the body and in males also serves as the conduit for semen.

23. **Scrotum** - The sac that contains the testes in males.

24. **Penis** - The male organ used for urination and sexual intercourse.

25. **Erection** - The process by which the penis becomes erect by engorging with blood.

26. **Ejaculation** - The discharge of semen from the male reproductive tract.

27. **Ovarian Cysts** - Fluid-filled sacs in an ovary or on its surface.

28. **Polycystic Ovary Syndrome (PCOS)** - A condition characterized by enlarged ovaries with small cysts on the outer edges.

29. **Hysterectomy** - Surgical removal of the uterus.

30. **Mastectomy** - Surgical removal of one or both breasts, partially or completely.

31. **Cesarean Section (C-Section)** - Surgical operation for delivering a child by cutting through the wall of the mother's abdomen.

32. **Pap Smear** - A test for cervical cancer in women, involving the collection of cells from the cervix.

33. **Mammography** - A technique using X-rays to diagnose and locate tumors of the breasts.

34. **Endometriosis** - A condition resulting from the appearance of endometrial tissue outside the uterus causing pelvic pain.

35. **Prostatitis** - Inflammation of the prostate gland.

36. **Vasectomy** - Surgical cutting and sealing of part of each vas deferens as a means of sterilization.

37. **Tubal Ligation** - A surgical procedure for female sterilization involving the blocking or sealing of the fallopian tubes.

38. **Intrauterine Device (IUD)** - A device inserted into the uterus to prevent pregnancy.

39. **Ectopic Pregnancy** - A pregnancy in which the fetus develops outside the uterus, typically in a fallopian tube.

40. **Gynecology** - The medical practice dealing with the health of the female reproductive system.

41. **Obstetrics** - The branch of medicine and surgery concerned with childbirth and the care of women giving birth.

42. **Spermatogenesis** - The process of sperm cell development.

43. **Oogenesis** - The creation of an ovum (egg cell).

44. **Libido** - Sexual desire.

45. **Dysmenorrhea** - Painful menstruation.

46. **Amenorrhea** - Absence of menstruation.

47. **Preeclampsia** - A condition in pregnancy characterized by high blood pressure, sometimes with fluidretention and proteinuria.

48. **Eclampsia** - A severe complication of pregnancy that produces seizures and coma.

49. **Gestational Diabetes** - Diabetes that develops during pregnancy.

50. **Cervical Dysplasia** - Abnormal growth of cells on the cervix, which could potentially lead to cervical cancer.

51. **Human Papillomavirus (HPV)** - A virus that can cause genital warts and cervical cancer.

52. **Breast Cancer** - A malignant tumor that starts from cells of the breast.

53. **Prostate Cancer** - Cancer of the prostate gland, seen commonly in older men.

54. **Testicular Cancer** - Cancer in the male organs that produce sperm and testosterone.

55. **Ovarian Cancer** - Cancer in the ovaries, part of the female reproductive system.

56. **Uterine Cancer** - Cancer involving the uterus.

57. **Vulvodynia** - Chronic pain or discomfort around the opening of the vagina.

58. **Pelvic Inflammatory Disease (PID)** - Infection of the female reproductive organs.

59. **Chlamydia** - A sexually transmitted infection caused by bacteria.

60. **Gonorrhea** - A sexually transmitted bacterial infection that may involve the genitals, mouth, or rectum.

61. **Syphilis** - A sexually transmitted infection caused by bacteria.

62. **Herpes Genitalis** - A sexually transmitted infection characterized by genital sores caused by the herpes simplex virus.

63. **AIDS (Acquired Immunodeficiency Syndrome)** - A disease caused by HIV where the immune system is severely damaged.

64. HIV (Human Immunodeficiency Virus) - The virus that causes AIDS.

65. **Genital Warts** - A sexually transmitted infection characterized by warts on the genital area.

66. **Infertility** - The inability to conceive after a year of regular intercourse without contraception.

67. **In Vitro Fertilization (IVF)** - A process by which an egg is fertilized by sperm outside the body.

68. **Sperm Count** - The total number of sperm cells per semen sample.

69. **Miscarriage** - The spontaneous loss of a fetus before the 20th week of pregnancy.

70. **Stillbirth** - The birth of a baby who is born without any signs of life at or after 24 weeks of pregnancy.

71. **Neonatology** - The branch of medicine that deals with the care of newborns.

72. **Postpartum Period** - The period following childbirth.

73. **Lactation** - Production and secretion of milk by the breasts.

74. **Breastfeeding** - Feeding an infant or young child with milk from a woman's breast.

75. **Contraception** - Methods or devices used to prevent pregnancy.

76. **Barrier Methods** - Contraceptive methods that block the sperm from reaching the egg, such as condoms and diaphragms.

77. **Hormonal Contraceptives** - Birth control methods that rely on hormones to prevent ovulation.

78. **Emergency Contraception** - Methods used to prevent pregnancy after unprotected intercourse.

79. **Sterilization** - Permanent methods of contraception that include vasectomy and tubal ligation.

80. **Sexual Dysfunction** - Problems experienced during any phase of the sexual response cycle preventing the individual or couple from experiencing satisfaction.

81. **Erectile Dysfunction** - The inability to get or keep an erection firm enough for sexual intercourse.

82. **Premature Ejaculation** - A condition in which a man ejaculates earlier during sexual intercourse than he or his partner would like.

83. **Benign Prostatic Hyperplasia (BPH)** - Enlargement of the prostate gland that can cause urinary problems.

84. **Prostate-specific Antigen (PSA)** - A protein produced by the prostate gland which is measured to screen for prostate cancer.

85. **Endometrial Biopsy** - A procedure to take a small tissue sample of the uterine lining for testing.

86. **Colposcopy** - A procedure to closely examine the cervix, vagina, and vulva for signs of disease.

87. **Molar Pregnancy** - An abnormal form of pregnancy in which a non-viable fertilized egg implants in the uterus and will fail to come to term.

88. **Perimenopause** - The transition period before menopause during which the production of reproductive hormones decreases and menstruation becomes irregular.

89. **Cryopreservation** - Freezing cells, tissue, or embryos in order to preserve them for future use.

90. **Semen Analysis** - An examination of semen sample to assess fertility in men.

91. **Laparoscopy** - A surgical diagnostic procedure used to examine the organs inside the abdomen.

92. **Oophorectomy** - Surgical removal of one or both ovaries.

93. **Vasovasostomy** - A surgery to reverse a vasectomy, reconnecting the cut segments of the vas deferens.

94. **Orchidectomy** - Surgical removal of one or both testicles.

95. **Cervical Cap** - A contraceptive device that fits over the cervix to block sperm from entering the uterus.

96. **Kegel Exercises** - Exercises to strengthen the pelvic floor muscles, which support the uterus, bladder, and bowel.

97. **Menopausal Hormone Therapy (MHT)** - Hormones given to alleviate the symptoms of menopause.

98. **Prolapsed Uterus** - A condition where the uterus falls down into or protrudes out of the vagina.

99. **Sexually Transmitted Diseases (STDs)** - Infections generally acquired by sexual contact.

100. **Genital Herpes** - A sexually transmitted infection caused by the herpes simplex virus.

101. **Pelvic Exam** - A physical examination of a woman's reproductive organs.

102. **Biopsy** - The removal of tissue from any part of the body to examine it for disease.

103. **Breast Ultrasound** - An imaging technique that uses sound waves to visualize the internal structures of the breast.

104. **Digital Rectal Exam (DRE)** - An examination in which a physician inserts a finger into the rectum to feel the texture, size, and shape of the prostate gland.

105. **Fibroids** - Noncancerous growths in the uterus that can develop during a woman's childbearing years.

106. **Papilloma** - A small, wart-like growth on the skin or on a mucous membrane, derived from the epidermis and usually benign.

107. **Vulvectomy** - Surgical removal of all or part of the vulva.

108. **Andropause** - A term used to describe decreased levels of testosterone in older men, comparable to menopause in women.

109. **Dilation and Curettage (D&C)** - A procedure to remove tissue from inside the uterus.

110. **Leiomyoma** - Another term for a fibroid, a benign tumor of the muscle layer of the uterus.

111. **Transvaginal Ultrasound** - An ultrasound performed with a transducer wand inserted in the vagina to get a closer and clearer view of the pelvic organs.

112. **Endometrial Ablation** - A procedure to destroy (ablate) the lining of the uterus (endometrium), which can reduce or stop menstrual flow.

113. **Ovarian Reserve Test** - A test used to determine the capacity of the ovary to provide egg cells that are capable of fertilization resulting in a healthy and successful pregnancy.

114. **Sperm Motility** - The ability of sperm to move efficiently, which is important for fertility.

115. **Sperm Morphology** - The size and shape of sperm, which is evaluated during semen analysis.

Endocrine System

1. **Endocrine System** - The system of glands that produce endocrine secretions that help to control bodily metabolic activity.

2. **Glands** - Organs in the body that secrete hormones.

3. **Hormones** - Chemical substances produced in the body that regulate the activity of cells or organs.

4. **Pituitary Gland** - The master gland of the endocrine system that controls other glands and makes several important hormones.

5. **Thyroid Gland** - A gland that makes hormones that regulate the way the body uses energy.

6. **Hypothalamus** - A section of the brain responsible for hormone production that controls body temperature, hunger, moods and the release of hormones from other glands.

7. **Adrenal Glands** - Glands that produce hormones such as adrenaline and cortisol.

8. **Pancreas** - A gland that makes insulin and glucagon, which help control blood sugar levels.

9. **Insulin** - A hormone produced by the pancreas that regulates blood sugar levels.

10. **Glucagon** - A hormone that raises blood glucose levels; the opposite of insulin.

11. **Parathyroid Glands** - Small glands of the endocrine system which regulate the calcium in our bodies.

12. **Calcitonin** - A hormone secreted by the thyroid that lowers blood calcium levels.

13. **Cortisol** - A steroid hormone produced by the adrenal cortex that regulates a wide range of processes throughout the body including metabolism and the immune response.

14. **Epinephrine (Adrenaline)** - A hormone secreted by the adrenal glands that increases rates of blood circulation, breathing, and carbohydrate metabolism and prepares muscles for exertion.

15. **Norepinephrine (Noradrenaline)** - A hormone that is important for attentiveness, emotions, sleeping, dreaming, and learning.

16. **Estrogen** - Female hormone produced by the ovaries; promotes female secondary sexual characteristics.

17. **Progesterone** - A hormone released by the ovaries that regulates the condition of the inner lining (endometrium) of the uterus.

18. **Testosterone** - The primary male sex hormone responsible for male sexual development and muscle mass.

19. **Growth Hormone (GH)** - Hormone secreted by the pituitary gland that stimulates growth of bones and muscle.

20. **Prolactin** - Hormone secreted by the pituitary gland that stimulates milk production.

21. **Oxytocin** - A hormone released by the pituitary gland that causes increased contraction of the uterus during labor and stimulates the ejection of milk into the ducts of the breasts.

22. **Antidiuretic Hormone (ADH)** - A hormone that helps the kidneys manage the amount of water in your body.

23. **Thyroxine (T4)** - A hormone which acts as a catalyst in the body for metabolism.

24. **Triiodothyronine (T3)** - Active thyroid hormone that regulates several metabolic processes including growth and energy expenditure.

25. **Melatonin** - A hormone that regulates sleep-wake cycles.

26. **Gonadotropins** - Hormones that stimulate the testes or ovaries.

27. **Leptin** - A hormone produced by fat cells that signals the brain to regulate appetite.

28. **Ghrelin** - A hormone produced in the stomach that stimulates hunger.

29. **Somatostatin** - A hormone that inhibits the secretion of several other hormones including growth hormone and insulin.

30. **Androgens** - Steroid hormones, such as testosterone, that control the development and maintenance of masculine characteristics.

31. **Catecholamines** - Hormones produced by the adrenal glands involved in the body's stress response.

32. **Aldosterone** - A hormone produced by the adrenal cortex that regulates salt and water balance.

33. **Corticosteroids** - Steroid hormones produced by the adrenal cortex.

34. **Endocrinology** - The branch of medicine concerned with the structure, function, and disorders of the endocrine glands.

35. **Follicle-Stimulating Hormone (FSH)** - A hormone involved in the development of eggs in women and sperm in men.

36. **Luteinizing Hormone (LH)** - A hormone that triggers ovulation and the development of the corpus luteum in females and stimulates testosterone production in males.

37. **Thyroid-Stimulating Hormone (TSH)** - A hormone produced by the pituitary gland that stimulates the thyroid gland to produce thyroid hormones.

38. **Pineal Gland** - A small gland in the brain that produces melatonin.

39. **Neuroendocrine Cells** - Cells that receive neuronal input and release message molecules (hormones) into the blood.

40. **Hormone Receptor** - A receptor molecule that binds hormones, initiating a cellular response.

41. **Negative Feedback** - A mechanism by which the body maintains homeostasis by reducing the output or activity of any organ or system back to its normal range of functioning.

42. **Positive Feedback** - A mechanism that enhances or amplifies changes; this tends to move a system away from its equilibrium state and make it more unstable.

43. **Hormonal Imbalance** - When there is too much or too little of a hormone in the bloodstream.

44. **Diabetes Mellitus** - A metabolic disorder characterized by high blood glucose levels due to insufficient insulin production or action.

45. **Hyperthyroidism** - Overactivity of the thyroid gland resulting in high levels of thyroid hormones and accelerated metabolism.

46. **Hypothyroidism** - Underactivity of the thyroid gland resulting in low levels of thyroid hormones.

47. **Cushing's Syndrome** - A condition caused by prolonged exposure to high levels of cortisol.

48. **Addison's Disease** - A disorder that occurs when the adrenal glands do not produce enough hormones.

49. **Gigantism** - A condition produced by hypersecretion of growth hormone during the early years of life.

50. **Acromegaly** - Enlargement of the extremities or limbs due to excessive secretion of growth hormone in adulthood.

51. **Pheochromocytoma** - A rare tumor of adrenal gland tissue that results in the release of too much epinephrine and norepinephrine.

52. **Polycystic Ovary Syndrome (PCOS)** - A condition in women characterized by irregular or no menstrual periods, acne, obesity, and excess hair growth.

53. **Menopause** - The time in a woman's life when her menstrual periods permanently stop and the body goes through changes that no longer allow her to get pregnant.

54. **Thyroid Nodule** - A growth (lump) in the thyroid gland.

55. **Thyroidectomy** - Surgical removal of all or part of the thyroid gland.

56. **Hyperparathyroidism** - Excessive production of parathyroid hormone by the parathyroid glands.

57. **Hypoparathyroidism** - Underproduction of parathyroid hormone, leading to low levels of calcium in the blood.

58. **Thyroid Cancer** - Cancer that forms in the thyroid gland.

59. **Endocrine Disruptors** - Chemicals that can interfere with endocrine systems at certain doses.

60. **Insulin Resistance** - A condition in which the body's cells become resistant to the effects of insulin.

61. **Metabolic Syndrome** - A cluster of conditions that increase the risk of heart disease, stroke, and diabetes.

62. **Goiter** - An abnormal enlargement of the thyroid gland.

63. **Exophthalmos** - Bulging of the eye anteriorly out of the orbit, often due to hyperthyroidism.

64. **Hirsutism** - Excessive hair growth on the face or body, particularly in women.

65. **Hypogonadism** - Decreased functional activity of the gonads, with associated reduction in the production of hormones.

66. **Ketoacidosis** - A serious diabetic complication where the body produces excess blood acids (ketones).

67. **Osteoporosis** - A condition where bones become weak and brittle, often due to hormonal imbalances affecting calcium absorption.

68. **Puberty** - The period during which adolescents reach sexual maturity and become capable of reproduction, regulated by hormonal changes.

69. **Reproductive Hormones** - Hormones that affect sexual functions and characteristics, such as estrogen, progesterone, and testosterone.

70. **Synthetic Hormones** - Man-made hormones used to treat certain medical conditions that mimic the effects of naturally occurring hormones.

71. **Thyroid Function Tests** - Blood tests used to measure how well the thyroid gland is working.

72. **Adrenocorticotropic Hormone (ACTH)** - A hormone produced by the pituitary gland that stimulates the adrenal glands.

73. **Calcium Homeostasis** - The regulation of calcium levels in the blood by the parathyroid hormone and calcitonin.

74. **Steroid Hormones** - Hormones that are synthesized from cholesterol and include testosterone, estrogens, and cortisol.

75. **Hormone Therapy** - Treatment using hormones to supplement a deficiency or adjust levels in the body, often used in menopause and cancer treatment.

76. **Pancreatectomy** - Surgical removal of all or part of the pancreas.

77. **Graves' Disease** - An autoimmune disorder that results in the overproduction of thyroid hormones (hyperthyroidism).

78. **Hashimoto's Thyroiditis** - An autoimmune disease in which the thyroid gland is gradually destroyed.

79. **Insulin Pump** - A medical device used to administer insulin in the treatment of diabetes.

80. **Glucose Tolerance Test** - A test to assess the body's ability to metabolize glucose, used in the diagnosis of diabetes.

81. **Bioidentical Hormones** - Man-made hormones that are chemically identical to those the human body produces.

82. **Neurosecretory Cells** - Cells in the nervous system that produce and release hormones.

83. **Circadian Rhythms** - Physical, mental, and behavioral changes that follow a 24-hour cycle, largely influenced by light and darkness in an organism's environment, often regulated by hormones.

84. **Endocrine Pancreas** - Part of the pancreas involved in producing and secreting hormones such as insulin and glucagon.

85. **Thyroid Peroxidase Antibodies (TPOAb)** - Antibodies that can attack the thyroid gland, often measured to diagnose thyroid autoimmune disorders.

86. **Somatotropic Cells** - Cells in the anterior pituitary gland that produce growth hormone.

87. **Dwarfism** - Condition of short stature as a result of a genetic or medical condition; often due to a deficiency in growth hormone.

88. **Gonadal Steroids** - Steroids produced by the gonads (ovaries or testes), including estrogen and testosterone.

89. **Adrenal Medulla** - The inner part of the adrenal gland that produces catecholamines, such as adrenaline.

90. **Hypophysis** - Another term for the pituitary gland.

91. **Incretins** - Hormones that decrease blood glucose levels by affecting the amount of insulin released after eating.

92. **Lipid Metabolism** - The process by which lipids are synthesized and degraded in the body, often influenced by hormones.

93. **Neuroendocrine Tumors** - Tumors that arise from cells that release hormones into the blood in response to a signal from the nervous system.

94. **Prolactinoma** - A benign tumor of the pituitary gland that produces a high level of prolactin.

95. **Secondary Hypothyroidism** - A form of hypothyroidism caused by failure of the pituitary gland to secrete thyroid-stimulating hormone (TSH).

96. **Thymus Gland** - A specialized organ of the immune system where T cells (T lymphocytes) mature, also involved in endocrine functions.

97. **Vasopressin** - Another name for antidiuretic hormone, which is involved in water balance and vasoconstriction.

98. **Zona Glomerulosa** - The outermost layer of the adrenal cortex that produces aldosterone.

99. **Zona Fasciculata** - The middle layer of the adrenal cortex that produces cortisol.

   a. **Zona Reticularis** - The innermost layer of the adrenal cortex that produces androgens.

100. **Estrogen Replacement Therapy (ERT)** - A treatment involving estrogen hormones to alleviate symptoms of menopause and reduce the risk of osteoporosis.

101. **Growth Hormone-Releasing Hormone (GHRH)** - A hormone produced by the hypothalamus that stimulates the pituitary gland to release growth hormone.

102. **Insulin-Like Growth Factor (IGF)** - A hormone similar in molecular structure to insulin, it plays an important role in childhood growth and continues to have anabolic effects in adults.

103. **Multiple Endocrine Neoplasia (MEN)** - A group of disorders that affect the endocrine system, leading to the development of tumors in multiple endocrine glands.

104. **Parathyroidectomy** - Surgical removal of one or more of the parathyroid glands, typically to treat hyperparathyroidism.

105. **Testosterone Replacement Therapy (TRT)** - A treatment intended to boost levels of testosterone in men with low levels due to aging or other conditions.

106. **Thyrotropin-Releasing Hormone (TRH)** - A hormone from the hypothalamus that stimulates the pituitary gland to release thyroid-stimulating hormone (TSH).

107. **Adrenalectomy** - Surgical removal of one or both adrenal glands.

108. **Corticotropin-Releasing Hormone (CRH)** - A hormone released by the hypothalamus that stimulates the pituitary gland to release adrenocorticotropic hormone (ACTH).

109. **DHEA (Dehydroepiandrosterone)** - A hormone produced by the adrenal glands that serves as a precursor to other hormones, including testosterone and estrogen.

110. **Euthyroid Sick Syndrome** - A condition in which thyroid function tests are abnormal in the setting of a non-thyroidal illness, without true dysfunction of the thyroid gland.

111. **Glucocorticoids** - A class of corticosteroids that play a role in glucose metabolism, immune function, and stress response.

112. **Mineralocorticoids** - A class of corticosteroids, such as aldosterone, that help control blood pressure and balance electrolytes.

113. **Pancreatic Polypeptide (PP)** - A hormone produced by the pancreas that helps regulate both the exocrine and endocrine functions of the pancreas.

114. **Somatostatin** - A hormone that inhibits the release of growth hormone and insulin.

Infectious Diseases

1. **Pathogen** - An organism that causes disease.

2. **Bacteria** - Single-celled microorganisms that can cause infections.

3. **Virus** - A microscopic infectious agent that replicates only inside the living cells of an organism.

4. **Fungi** - A kingdom of usually multicellular, eukaryotic organisms that can cause infections.

5. **Protozoa** - Single-celled eukaryotes that can cause parasitic diseases.

6. **Helminths** - Parasitic worms that cause disease and illness.

7. **Prion** - Infectious agents composed entirely of protein material that can fold in multiple, structurally abnormal ways.

8. **Epidemic** - A widespread occurrence of an infectious disease in a community at a particular time.

9. **Pandemic** - An epidemic of a disease that has spread across a large region, for instance multiple continents or worldwide.

10. **Endemic** - A disease or condition regularly found among particular people or in a certain area.

11. **Antibiotics** - Drugs used to fight bacterial infections.

12. **Antivirals** - Medications that treat viral infections.

13. **Antifungals** - Drugs that specifically target fungal infections.

14. **Antiparasitics** - Medications used to treat infections caused by parasites.

15. **Vaccine** - A biological preparation that provides active acquired immunity to a particular infectious disease.

16. **Immunization** - The process whereby a person is made immune or resistant to an infectious disease, typically by the administration of a vaccine.

17. **Incubation Period** - The period between exposure to an infection and the appearance of the first symptoms.

18. **Contagious** - Capable of being transmitted from one individual to another through direct or indirect contact.

19. **Transmission** - The way a pathogen is spread from one host to another.

20. **Vector** - An organism, typically a biting insect or tick, that transmits a disease or parasite from one animal or plant to another.

21. **Zoonosis** - An infectious disease that has passed from an animal to humans.

22. **Reservoir** - The primary habitat in which a pathogen lives, grows, and multiplies.

23. **Carrier** - A person or organism that has contracted an infectious disease but displays no symptoms.

24. **Outbreak** - A sudden rise in the incidence of a disease.

25. **Morbidity** - The condition of being diseased or the incidence of disease within a population.

26. **Mortality** - The state of being mortal; often used to refer to the number of deaths caused by a disease in a population.

27. **Nosocomial Infection** - An infection acquired in a hospital setting.

28. **Infection Control** - Practices implemented in healthcare settings to prevent the spread of infectious diseases.

29. **Quarantine** - Restricting the movement of people or goods to prevent the spread of disease.

30. **Isolation** - Separating individuals who are ill from those who are healthy to prevent the spread of infectious diseases.

31. **Pathogenicity** - The ability of an organism to cause disease.

32. **Virulence** - The degree of pathogenicity within a group or species of parasites as indicated by case fatality rates.

33. **Epidemiology** - The study and analysis of the distribution, patterns, and determinants of health and disease conditions in defined populations.

34. **Microbiology** - The study of microscopic organisms, such as bacteria, viruses, archaea, fungi, and protozoa.

35. **Serology** - The study of serum and other bodily fluids, which is often used to diagnose infections by the detection of antibodies or antigens.

36. **Culture** - The propagation of microorganisms or cells in a growth medium.

37. **Sensitivity Testing** - Tests used to determine the "sensitivity" of bacteria to an antibiotic.

38. **Gram Stain** - A method of staining used to distinguish and classify bacterial species into two large groups (gram-positive and gram-negative).

39. **Immunodeficiency** - A state in which the immune system's ability to fight infectious disease is compromised or entirely absent.

40. **Disinfection** - The process of cleaning something, especially with a chemical, in order to destroy bacteria.

41. **Sterilization** - Any process that eliminates, removes, kills, or deactivates all forms of life and other biological agents.

42. **Prophylaxis** - Action taken to prevent disease, especially by specified means or against a specified disease.

43. **Incidence** - The occurrence, rate, or frequency of a disease.

44. **Prevalence** -The total number of cases of a disease in a population at a given time.

45. **Asymptomatic** - Showing no symptoms of disease.

46. **Symptomatic** - Showing symptoms of disease.

47. **Invasive Disease** - An infection that enters the body and affects internal organs.

48. **Non-invasive Disease** - Disease that does not enter the body beyond the site of initial contact.

49. **Latent Infection** - Infection with a pathogen that lies dormant but can become active.

50. **Acute Infection** - An infection of short duration that is often severe.

51. **Chronic Infection** - An infection that persists over a long period of time.

52. **Subclinical Infection** - An infection that stays below the surface of clinical detection.

53. **Secondary Infection** - An infection that occurs during or after treatment for another infection.

54. **Opportunistic Infection** - An infection caused by pathogens that take advantage of an opportunity not normally available, such as a weakened immune system.

55. **Hereditary Disease** - Disease caused by mutation that is passed from one generation to another.

56. **Congenital Disease** - Disease that is present at birth.

57. **Vector-borne Disease** - Disease transmitted by a vector, such as mosquitoes, ticks, or flies.

58. **Foodborne Illness** - Illness caused by food contaminated with bacteria, viruses, parasites, or toxins.

59. **Waterborne Disease** - Diseases caused by pathogenic microorganisms that most commonly are transmitted in contaminated fresh water.

60. **Aerosol Transmission** - Transmission of an infectious agent by airborne droplets.

61. **Fomite Transmission** - The transmission of infectious diseases by objects, or fomites, which carry infection from one individual to another.

62. **Direct Contact Transmission** - The transfer of an infectious agent from one individual to another through direct physical contact.

63. **Indirect Contact Transmission** - The transfer of pathogens via an intermediate object or person.

64. **Droplet Transmission** - A mode of transmission for pathogens spread through large respiratory droplets expelled by the infectious agent.

65. **Vertical Transmission** - Transmission of a pathogen from a mother to her baby during the period immediately before and after birth.

66. **Horizontal Transmission** - The transmission of infections between members of the same species that are not in a parent-child relationship.

67. **Incidental Host** - A host that generally does not allow transmission of the pathogen to other hosts.

68. **Definitive Host** - An organism that supports the adult or sexually reproductive form of a parasite.

69. **Intermediate Host** - An organism that supports the immature or non-reproductive forms of a parasite.

70. **Reinfection** - The process of being infected again with the same pathogen after recovery.

71. **Cross-Immunity** - Immunity to one agent that provides immunity to another related agent.

72. **Herd Immunity** - Resistance to the spread of a contagious disease within a population that results if a sufficiently high proportion of individuals are immune to the disease, especially through vaccination.

73. **Passive Immunity** - The short-term immunity that results from the introduction of antibodies from another person or animal.

74. **Active Immunity** - Protection that is produced by a person's own immune system and usually lasts a lifetime.

75. **Booster Shot** - An additional dose of a vaccine needed periodically to 'boost' the immune system.

76. **Live Attenuated Vaccine** - A vaccine made from a pathogen that has been weakened but still alive.

77. **Inactivated Vaccine** - A vaccine made from a pathogen that has been killed or inactivated.

78. **Subunit Vaccine** - A vaccine that includes only parts of the virus or bacteria.

79. **Toxoid Vaccine** - A vaccine made from a toxin (poison) that has been made harmless but that elicits an immune response against the toxin.

80. **DNA Vaccine** - A vaccine that uses genetically engineered DNA to induce an immune response.

81. **RNA Vaccine** - A vaccine that uses mRNA to instruct cells how to make a protein that will prompt an immune response.

82. **Adjuvant** - A substance that enhances the body's immune response to an antigen.

83. **Public Health** - The science and art of preventing disease, prolonging life, and promoting health through organized efforts and informed choices of society, organizations, public and private communities, and individuals.

84. **Outbreak Investigation** - The process of reviewing the spread of disease to pinpoint its source and how it spreads.

85. **Case Definition** - A standard criterion for classifying whether a person has a particular disease, syndrome, or other health condition.

86. **Case Fatality Rate** - The proportion of people who die from a specified disease among all individuals diagnosed with the disease.

87. **Contact Tracing** - The process of identifying, assessing, and managing people who have been exposed to a disease to prevent onward transmission.

88. **Surveillance** - Continuous, systematic collection, analysis, and interpretation of health-related data needed for the planning, implementation, and evaluation of public health practice.

89. **Syndromic Surveillance** - Surveillance using health-related data that precedes diagnosis and signals a sufficient probability of a case or an outbreak to warrant further public health response.

90. **Biological Warfare** - The use of biological toxins or infectious agents such as bacteria, viruses, and fungi with the intent to kill or incapacitate humans, animals, or plants as an act of war.

91. **Biodefense** - Any means used to restore biosecurity to a group of organisms who are, or may be, subject to biological threats or infectious diseases.

92. **PPE (Personal Protective Equipment)** - Equipment worn to minimize exposure to hazards that cause serious workplace injuries and illnesses.

93. **Sanitation** - The development and application of sanitary measures for the sake of cleanliness, protecting health, etc.

94. **Disinfectant** - A chemical liquid that destroys bacteria.

95. **Pandemic Preparedness** - Activities and measures taken beforehand to prepare and possibly prevent the outbreak of a pandemic.

96. **Eradication** - The complete and permanent worldwide reduction to zero new cases of an infectious disease through deliberate efforts; no further control measures required.

97. **Elimination** - Reduction to zero of the incidence of a specified disease in a defined geographic area as a result of deliberate efforts; continued measures to prevent re-establishment of transmission are required.

98. **Quarantine Measures** - Health measures, such as isolation and observation, applied to individuals to prevent the spread of disease.

99. **Viral Load** - The number of virus particles in a specific volume of fluid; commonly used in reference to HIV or hepatitis C.

100. **Mutation** - The changing of the structure of a gene, resulting in a variant form that may be transmitted to subsequent generations.

101. **Genetic Variation** - Differences in DNA among individuals or populations.

102. **Host** - An organism that harbors a virus or parasite.

103. **Microbiota** - The microorganisms of a particular site, habitat, or geological period.

104.   **Flora** - In a medical context, this refers to the microbial community found on or in a healthy person.

105.   **Superinfection** - An infection following a previous infection especially when caused by microorganisms that are resistant or have become resistant to the antibiotics used earlier.

106.   **Antimicrobial Resistance (AMR)** - The ability of a microbe to resist the effects of medication previously used to treat them.

107.   **Broad-Spectrum Antibiotics** - Antibiotics that act on the two major bacterial groups, Gram-positive and Gram-negative, or on many species of bacteria.

108.   **Narrow-Spectrum Antibiotics** - Antibiotics that are effective against specific families of bacteria.

109.   **Probiotics** - Live microorganisms intended to provide health benefits when consumed, generally by improving or restoring the gut flora.

110.   **Bacteriostatic** - A biological or chemical agent that stops bacteria from reproducing, while not necessarily killing them otherwise.

111.   **Bactericidal** - A substance that kills bacteria.

112.   **Virology** - The study of viruses and viral diseases.

113.   **Mycology** - The branch of biology concerned with the study of fungi, including their genetic and biochemical properties.

114.   **Parasitology** - The study of parasites, their hosts, and the relationship between them.

115.   **Immunocompromised** - Having an impaired immune system, which decreases the ability to fight infections and other diseases.

Oncological Terminology

1. **Oncology** - The branch of medicine that specializes in the diagnosis and treatment of cancer.

2. **Carcinoma** - A type of cancer that starts in the cells that make up the skin or the tissue lining organs, such as the liver or kidneys.

3. **Sarcoma** - A type of cancer that originates from connective tissues such as bone, muscle, fat, or cartilage.

4. **Leukemia** - A type of cancer found in blood and bone marrow, characterized by the rapid production of abnormal white blood cells.

5. **Lymphoma** - A group of blood cancers that develop from lymphocytes, a type of white blood cell.

6. **Metastasis** - The spread of cancer cells from the place where they first formed to another part of the body.

7. **Benign** - A tumor that is not cancerous and does not spread to nearby tissues or other parts of the body.

8. **Malignant** - A cancerous tumor that can invade and destroy nearby tissue and spread to other parts of the body.

9. **Biopsy** - A medical test involving the removal of cells or tissues for examination to determine the presence of cancer.

10. **Chemotherapy** - A type of cancer treatment that uses drugs to kill cancer cells.

11. **Radiation Therapy** - A treatment that uses high doses of radiation to kill cancer cells and shrink tumors.

12. **Immunotherapy** - A type of cancer treatment that helps your immune system fight cancer.

13. **Hormone Therapy** - Treatment that adds, blocks, or removes hormones to slow or stop the growth of cancer cells that use hormones to grow.

14. **Targeted Therapy** - A cancer treatment that uses drugs or other substances to precisely identify and attack cancer cells, usually while doing little damage to normal cells.

15. **Oncogene** - A gene that has the potential to cause cancer.

16. **Tumor Suppressor Genes** - Genes that protect a cell from one step on the path to cancer.

17. **Carcinogen** - Any substance that promotes carcinogenesis, the formation of cancer.

18. **Adjuvant Therapy** - Additional cancer treatment given after the primary treatment to lower the risk that the cancer will come back.

19. **Neoadjuvant Therapy** - Treatment given as a first step to shrink a tumor before the main treatment, which is usually surgery, is given.

20. **Palliative Care** - Specialized medical care that focuses on providing relief from pain and other symptoms of a serious illness.

21. **Oncologist** - A doctor who specializes in treating cancer.

22. **Pathologist** - A doctor who interprets and diagnoses the changes caused by disease in tissues and body fluids.

23. **Radiologist** - A doctor who uses medical imaging techniques to diagnose and treat diseases.

24. **Complete Response** - The disappearance of all signs of cancer in response to treatment.

25. **Partial Response** - A decrease in the size of a tumor, or in the extent of cancer in the body, in response to treatment.

26. **Progression-Free Survival** - The length of time during and after treatment that a patient lives with the disease without it getting worse.

27. **Overall Survival** - The length of time from either the date of diagnosis or the start of treatment for a disease, such as cancer, that patients diagnosed with the disease are still alive.

28. **Clinical Trial** - A research study that tests new medical approaches in people.

29. **Protocol** - A detailed plan of a scientific or medical experiment, treatment, or procedure.

30. **Stage** - A way of describing where the cancer is located, if or where it has spread, and whether it is affecting the functions of other organs in the body.

31. **Grade** - A scoring system used to describe the appearance of cancer cells and how quickly the tumor is likely to grow and spread.

32. **Remission** - A decrease or disappearance of signs and symptoms of cancer.

33. **Relapse** - The return of cancer after treatment and after a period of time in which the cancer could not be detected.

34. **Molecular Testing** - Tests done to identify specific genes, proteins, and other factors involved in the growth and spread of cancer.

35. **Personalized Medicine** - A form of medicine that uses information about a person's genes, proteins, and environment to prevent, diagnose, and treat disease.

36. **Biomarker** - A biological molecule found in blood, other body fluids, or tissues that is a sign of a normal or abnormal process, or of a condition or disease.

37. **Radiosurgery** - A treatment method that uses focused beams of high-dose radiation to treat small areas, often in the brain or spine, without making an actual incision.

38. **Cytotoxic** - Agents that are toxic to cells, preventing their replication or causing cell death.

39. **In situ** - Refers to cancer that has not spread from the original tissue.

40. **Invasive Cancer** - Cancer that has spread beyond the layer of tissue in which it developed and is growing into surrounding, healthy tissues.

41. **Laparoscopy** - A surgical diagnostic procedure used to examine the organs inside the abdomen with minimal incisions.

42. **Endoscopic Surgery** - A surgical technique using an endoscope to examine the interior of a hollow organ or cavity of the body.

43. **Brachytherapy** - A form of radiotherapy where a sealed radiation source is placed inside or next to the area requiring treatment.

44. **Cancer Screening** - Tests performed on individuals with no cancer symptoms to detect cancerous cells at an early stage.

45. **Prognosis** - The likely course and outcome of a disease, including the chances of recovery.

46. **Tumor Marker** - Substances, often proteins, produced by cancer cells or by the body in response to cancer, which can be found in the blood, urine, or tissues.

47. **Recurrence** - The return of cancer after treatment and after a period of time during which the cancer was undetected.

48. **Second Opinion** - Seeking advice from another doctor to confirm a diagnosis and evaluate treatment options.

49. **Supportive Care** - Treatments and medications that help alleviate symptoms, improve quality of life, and manage pain and other complications.

50. **Cytology** - The study of cells, including their function, structure, and life history, which is often used to diagnose cancer.

51. **Histology** - The study of the microscopic structure of tissues, often used to diagnose and differentiate cancer types.

52. **Oncolytic Virus Therapy** - A treatment that uses genetically modified viruses that selectively infect and kill cancer cells.

53. **Angiogenesis Inhibitors** - Drugs that prevent the growth of new blood vessels that tumors need to grow.

54. **Cancer Genomics** - The study of the totality of DNA sequence and gene expression differences between cancer cells and normal host cells.

55. **Epigenetics** - The study of biological mechanisms that will switch genes on and off in cancer.

56. **Radiomics** - The extraction of large amounts of features from radiographic medical images using data-characterization algorithms.

57. **Thermal Ablation** - Techniques that use extreme temperatures to destroy cancer cells, including radiofrequency, microwave, and cryoablation.

58. **Excision** - Surgical removal of part of a cancerous tissue.

59. **Margin** - The border or edge of a tissue removed during cancer surgery; examined to determine if cancer cells are present.

60. **Sentinel Lymph Node Biopsy** - A surgical procedure to determine if cancer has spread beyond a primary tumor into the lymphatic system.

61. **Lymphedema** - Swelling due to lymphatic fluid that occurs when lymph nodes are damaged or removed as part of cancer treatment.

62. **Pap Test** - A procedure to collect cells from the surface of the cervix or vagina to check for abnormalities that may be indicative of cervical cancer.

63. **Mammography** - An X-ray picture of the breast used to detect breast cancer.

64. **Bone Marrow Aspiration** - A procedure that involves taking a sample of the liquid part of the marrow to test for cancer cells.

65. **Bone Marrow Biopsy** - The removal of a small amount of solid tissue from bone marrow to examine under a microscope for signs of cancer.

66. **Stem Cell Transplant** - A procedure that restores blood-forming stem cells in cancer patients who have had theirs destroyed by very high doses of chemotherapy or radiation therapy.

67. **Cancer Fatigue** - A common and often debilitating symptom of cancer and cancer treatment that affects daily life.

68. **Dysplasia** - An abnormal type of cell growth that can be precancerous.

69. **Cryotherapy** - Treatment that uses extreme cold, often liquid nitrogen, to freeze and destroy abnormal tissue.

70. **Gene Therapy** - Techniques that modify a person's genes to treat or cure disease, including cancer.

71. **Photodynamic Therapy (PDT)** - A treatment that uses special drugs, called photosensitizing agents, alongside light to kill cancer cells.

72. **Anaplasia** - A condition of cells in which they have lost mature features and organization, often a characteristic of malignancy.

73. **Apoptosis** - The process of programmed cell death that occurs in multicellular organisms, often disrupted in cancer cells.

74. **Cachexia** - A complex metabolic syndrome associated with underlying illness and characterized by loss of muscle with or without loss of fat mass.

75. **Carcinoembryonic Antigen (CEA)** - A set of proteins found in some types of cancers and in lower amounts in normal tissue; used as a tumor marker.

76. **Combination Therapy** - Use of more than one medical treatment (e.g., surgery, radiation, chemotherapy) simultaneously or sequentially to maximize effectiveness.

77. **Computed Tomography (CT Scan)** - A diagnostic imaging procedure that uses a combination of X-rays and computer technology to produce horizontal, or axial, images of the body.

78. **Cytostatic** - Agents or drugs that inhibit cell growth and multiplication.

79. **Debulking Surgery** - Surgical removal of as much of a tumor as possible, typically used when complete resection is impossible.

80. **Differentiation** - How much or how little tumor tissue resembles the normal tissue from which it arose.

81. **Electrochemotherapy** - A treatment combining chemotherapy and electric pulses to increase the absorption of the chemotherapy drug by cancer cells.

82. **End-of-Life Care** - Support and medical care given during the time surrounding death.

83. **Enzyme Inhibitor Therapy** - A treatment strategy involving the use of drugs or agents to block the activity of enzymes that promote cancer cell growth and survival.

84. **Epidemiology** - The study of the distribution and determinants of health-related states or events in specified populations.

85. **Ewing Sarcoma** - A rare type of cancer occurring in the bones or in the soft tissue around the bones.

86. **Extravasation** - The leakage of intravenously (IV) infused, potentially damaging medications into the extravascular tissue around the site of infusion.

87. **Fibrosarcoma** - A malignant tumor composed of fibrous or connective tissue.

88. **Gastrointestinal Stromal Tumor (GIST)** - A type of tumor that occurs in the digestive tract, most commonly in the stomach or small intestine.

89. **Gene Expression Profiling** - A method used to analyze the types and amounts of mRNA transcripts present in a cell or tissue sample.

90. **Genetic Susceptibility** - Increased likelihood of developing a particular disease based on a person's genetic makeup.

91. **Gleason Score** - A system of grading prostate cancer tissue based on how it looks under a microscope.

92. **Hematologist** - A medical specialist who deals with diseases of the blood and blood-forming organs.

93. **Hepatocellular Carcinoma** - The most common type of liver cancer.

94. **HER2/neu** - A protein that can appear at high levels on some types of cancer cells, including breast and ovarian cancers.

95. **Hodgkin's Lymphoma** - A type of lymphoma characterized by the presence of Reed-Sternberg cells.

96. **Hyperplasia** - An increase in the number of cells in a tissue or organ, which can be a precursor of cancer.

97. **Idiopathic** - Relating to or denoting any disease or condition which arises spontaneously or for which the cause is unknown.

98. **Immunohistochemistry** - A laboratory method that uses antibodies to check for certain antigens (markers) in a sample of tissue.

99. **Intraoperative Radiation Therapy (IORT)** - A treatment during which radiation is delivered directly to the tumor site during surgery, minimizing exposure to surrounding normal tissue.

100. **Kaposi's Sarcoma** - A type of cancer that forms in the lining of blood and lymph vessels.

101. **Karyotype** - The number and appearance of chromosomes in the nucleus of a eukaryotic cell.

102. **Keratinizing** - The process by which epithelial cells become filled with keratin protein filaments, die, and form tough, resistant structures in the skin or mucous membranes.

103. **Laser Therapy** - The use of lasers to treat various medical conditions, including tumors, by cutting, burning, or destroying tissue.

104. **Leiomyosarcoma** - A rare type of cancer that originates in smooth muscle cells.

105. **Melanoma** - A type of skin cancer that begins in cells known as melanocytes.

106. **Mesothelioma** - A rare, aggressive form of cancer that primarily affects the lining of the lungs or abdomen, often associated with asbestos exposure.

107. **Metaplasia** - A reversible change from one type of cell to another type, often as an adaptation to a persistent stressor, which can sometimes lead to cancerous transformations.

108.   **Metastasis** - The process by which cancer cells spread from the place where they first formed to another part of the body.

109.   **Monoclonal Antibodies** - Lab-made proteins that can bind to substances in the body, including cancer cells; used in some types of targeted cancer therapy.

110.   **MRI (Magnetic Resonance Imaging)** - A medical imaging technique used in radiology to form pictures of the anatomy and the physiological processes of the body.

111.   **Myeloma** - A type of cancer that forms in plasma cells, which are a type of white blood cell made in the bone marrow.

112.   **Necrosis** - The death of cells or tissues through injury or disease, which can be a feature in tumors.

113.   **Neoadjuvant Therapy** - Treatment given as a first step to shrink a tumor before the main treatment, usually surgery, is done.

114.   **Neoplasm** - Another term for a tumor, which may be benign or malignant.

115.   **Nephrectomy** - Surgical removal of a kidney, often performed to treat kidney cancer.

Pharmacology

1. **Absorption** - The process by which drugs enter the bloodstream.

2. **Bioavailability** - The proportion of a drug that enters the circulation when introduced into the body and is able to have an active effect.

3. **Biotransformation** - The chemical modification made by an organism on a chemical compound.

4. **Catabolism** - The breakdown of drugs and other substances within the body.

5. **Contraindication** - A specific situation in which a drug, procedure, or surgery should not be used because it may be harmful to the person.

6. **Cytochrome P450** - A group of enzymes involved in drug metabolism and detoxification.

7. **Dosage Form** - The physical form of a dose of medication, such as a capsule, injection, or liquid.

8. **Drug Interaction** - A reaction between two (or more) drugs or between a drug and a food/beverage or supplement.

9. **Efficacy** - The ability of a drug to produce the desired therapeutic effect.

10. **Elimination** - The removal of drugs from the body, either in an unchanged form or as metabolites.

11. **Enteral Administration** - Drug delivery that uses the gastrointestinal tract, such as oral or rectal administration.

12. **Enzyme Induction** - The increase in enzyme activity that results in greater metabolism of drugs.

13. **Excretion** - The process of removing waste products and drugs from the body, typically through the kidneys.

14. **Half-Life** - The time it takes for the plasma concentration of a drug to reduce by half.

15. **Intravenous (IV)** - Administration of a substance directly into a vein.

16. **Ligand** - A substance that forms a complex with a biomolecule to serve a biological purpose, often a drug.

17. **Metabolite** - A product of metabolism; often refers to the breakdown products of drugs in the body.

18. **Nephrotoxicity** - Toxicity to the kidneys, often caused by drugs or toxins.

19. **Oral Bioavailability** - The proportion of an orally administered dose of a drug that reaches the systemic circulation.

20. **Pharmacodynamics** - The study of what a drug does to the body.

21. **Pharmacogenetics** - The study of how genetic variations affect an individual's response to drugs.

22. **Pharmacokinetics** - The study of how drugs move through the body.

23. **Placebo** - A substance with no therapeutic effect, used as a control in testing new drugs.

24. **Potency** - The amount of drug needed to produce a given effect.

25. **Prodrug** - A medication or compound that, after administration, is metabolized into a pharmacologically active drug.

26. **Receptor** - A molecule in a cell or on its surface that binds to a specific substance and causes a specific physiological effect.

27. **Side Effect** - An unwanted or unexpected effect caused by a drug.

28. **Sublingual Administration** - Placement of a drug under the tongue where it dissolves and is absorbed into the bloodstream.

29. **Synergism** - The interaction between drugs that causes their combined effect to be greater than the sum of their separate effects.

30. **Therapeutic Index** - The ratio between the toxic and therapeutic concentrations of a drug.

31. **Tolerance** - A reduced response to a drug after repeated use.

32. **Topical Administration** - Application of a drug directly to a body surface.

33. **Toxicology** - The study of the harmful effects of substances on living organisms.

34. **Volume of Distribution (Vd)** - A pharmacokinetic parameter that describes the distribution of a drug between plasma and the rest of the body.

35. **Withdrawal** - Symptoms that occur after stopping or reducing intake of a drug to which one has become addicted or tolerant.

36. **Xenobiotic** - A chemical substance that is foreign to the biological system.

37. **Zero-Order Kinetics** - Drug elimination with a constant amount metabolized regardless of drug concentration.

38. **Agonist** - A substance that activates a receptor to produce a biological response.

39. **Antagonist** - A substance that blocks or dampens agonist-mediated responses.

40. **Bioequivalence** - A term in pharmacokinetics that indicates that two drugs release their active ingredient into the bloodstream at the same rate and to the same extent.

41. **Chelation** - A type of bonding of ions and molecules to metal ions and used in some drugs to enhance their stability or to reduce toxicity.

42. **Clinical Trial** - A research study that tests how well new medical approaches work in people.

43. **Compliance (Adherence)** - The extent to which a patient correctly follows medical advice.

44. **Dose-response Relationship** - The relationship between the quantity of a drug given and its effect on the body.

45. **Drug Delivery System** - Technology used to deliver drugs or chemical substances in the body.

46. **Drug Resistance** - Reduction in effectiveness of a drug such as an antimicrobial or an antineoplastic in curing a disease or condition.

47. **First-pass Metabolism** - The phenomenon of drug metabolism whereby the concentration of a drug is greatly reduced before it reaches the systemic circulation.

48. **Generic Drug** - A drug that has the same chemical substance as a drug that was originally protected by chemical patents.

49. **Hepatotoxicity** - Liver toxicity, often caused by drugs or toxins.

50. **Idiosyncratic Reaction** - An uncommon response to a drug that is unpredictable and not due to dose or duration of administration.

51. **Inhalation Administration** - Delivery of drugs through the respiratory tract by inhalers or nebulizers.

52. **Intramuscular (IM)** - Administration of a substance directly into a muscle.

53. **Local Effect** - A response to a medication that occurs at the site of application.

54. **Maintenance Dose** - The dosage of a drug required to keep the drug blood level at a steady state in order to maintain the desired effect.

55. **Mechanism of Action** - The specific biochemical interaction through which a drug substance produces its pharmacological effect.

56. **Nocebo Effect** - A detrimental effect on health produced by psychological or psychosomatic factors such as negative expectations of treatment or prognosis.

57. **Off-Label Use** - The use of pharmaceutical drugs for an unapproved indication or in an unapproved age group, dosage, or route of administration.

58. **Overdose** - Taking an excessive amount of a drug leading to severe adverse reactions.

59. **Pharmacoeconomics** - The study of the economic implications of drug therapy, including costs and benefits.

60. **Pharmacovigilance** - The science and activities relating to the detection, assessment, understanding, and prevention of adverse effects or any other drug-related problem.

61. **Prophylactic Therapy** - Treatment given or action taken to prevent disease.

62. **Rectal Administration** - Drug delivery route where the drug is inserted into the rectum.

63. **Selective Toxicity** - The ability of a drug to target sites that are relatively specific to the microorganism responsible for infection or to neoplastic cells.

64. **Serum Sickness** - An immune system reaction to certain medications causing symptoms like rash, fever, and joint pain.

65. **Subcutaneous Administration** - Administration of a substance into the layer of skin directly below the dermis and epidermis, collectively referred to as the cutaneous layer.

66. **Titration** - The process of gradually adjusting the dose of a medication until the desired effect is achieved.

67. **Transdermal Patch** - A medicated adhesive patch placed on the skin to deliver a specific dose of medication through the skin and into the bloodstream.

68. **Vehicle** - The substance in which a drug is delivered, such as a capsule, tablet, or liquid.

69. **Vesicant** - A chemical that causes extensive tissue damage and blistering upon contact.

70. **Zoonosis** - Any disease or infection that is naturally transmissible from vertebrate animals to humans.

71. **Analgesic** - A type of medication used to relieve pain.

72. **Anxiolytic** - A drug that helps reduce anxiety.

73. **Autonomic Nervous System** - Part of the nervous system that controls involuntary bodily functions and is a target for some pharmacological agents.

74. **Bioinformatics** - The application of computer technology to the management of biological information, often used in drug design.

75. **Blinded Study** - A study in which participants are unaware of whether they are receiving the experimental drug, the standard treatment, or a placebo.

76. **Buccal Administration** - Drug delivery through the mucous membrane lining the cheek.

77. **Carcinogenicity** - The potential of a substance to cause cancer.

78. **Cross-sensitivity** - A condition where a person allergic to a particular drug also shows an allergy to another, structurally similar drug.

79. **Cytostatic** - A drug or agent that inhibits cell growth and multiplication.

80. **Depot Injection** - A method of administering medications in a vehicle that allows gradual release of the medication to maintain a constant drug concentration.

81. **Dissolution** - The process by which a drug goes into solution in the body and becomes available for absorption.

82. **Double-blind Study** - A study in which neither the participants nor the experimenters know who is receiving a particular treatment.

83. **Drug Formulary** - A list of prescription medications approved for use by a health plan or hospital.

84. **Emetic** - A substance that induces vomiting.

85. **Endocrine System** - A system of glands that produce hormones, often targeted by hormone therapies or other drugs.

86. **Excipient** - An inactive substance formulated alongside the active ingredient of a medication for the purpose of bulking-up formulations that contain potent active ingredients.

87. **Fixed-dose Combination (FDC)** - A medication that contains two or more active ingredients combined in a single dosage form.

88. **Gastric Emptying** - The process by which food leaves the stomach and enters the small intestine, important in the timing of medication absorption.

89. **Hormone Replacement Therapy (HRT)** - The use of the female hormones estrogen and progestin (a synthetic form of progesterone) to replace those the body no longer makes after menopause.

90. **Inotropic Agent** - A drug that alters the force or energy of muscular contractions, particularly in the heart.

91. **Lipophilicity** - The chemical property of being fat soluble, which influences how drugs are absorbed, distributed, and enter the brain.

92. **Loading Dose** - A higher dose of a drug given at the beginning of a course of treatment to rapidly achieve a therapeutic level.

93. **Mucolytic** - A drug that helps break down mucus so it is easier to clear from the airways.

94. **Neurotransmitter** - A chemical that transmits signals across a chemical synapse, such as between a neuron and a muscle or between two neurons.

95. **Ophthalmic Administration** - Drug delivery directly into the eye.

96. **Pharmacopoeia** - An official publication containing a list of medicinal drugs with their effects and directions for their use.

97. **Placebo-Controlled Study** - A study that compares the effects of a drug with a placebo.

98. **Polypharmacy** - The use of multiple medications by a patient, typically an older adult, which can increase the risk of adverse effects and drug interactions.

99. **Preservative** - A substance added to medications to prevent microbial growth.

100. **Randomized Controlled Trial (RCT)** - A clinical study where participants are randomly assigned to receive one of the clinical interventions under study.

101. **Reuptake Inhibitor** - A substance that increases the level of neurotransmitters in the brain by blocking their absorption.

102. **Sedative** - A substance that induces sedation by reducing irritability or excitement.

103. **Substrate** - A substance on which an enzyme acts.

104. **Therapeutic Window** - The range of drug doses which can treat disease effectively while staying within the safety range.

105. **Vasoconstrictor** - A drug that causes the narrowing of the blood vessels, thereby decreasing blood flow.

106. **Vasodilator** - A drug that causes blood vessels to widen, increasing blood flow.

107. **Water-soluble** - Able to dissolve in water, significant for how drugs are formulated and administered.

108. **Withdrawal Trial** - A trial where the drug is ceased to see if the patient relapses, used to assess efficacy and dependency.

109. **Xenograft** - A transplant of tissue from one species to another, often used in research to study the effects of drugs on human tissues.

110. **Yield** - The amount of active drug or chemical produced from a specific process, important in pharmaceutical manufacturing for efficacy and cost-effectiveness.

111. **Antipyretic** - A type of medication used to prevent or reduce fever.

112. **Biologic** - A type of drug derived from living organisms through biotechnology; includes a wide range of products such as vaccines, blood components, or antibodies.

113. **Chronotherapy** - The strategy of administering medications in coordination with the body's clock, aiming to optimize effectiveness and reduce side effects.

114. **Dermatological Agent** - A drug that is used for the treatment of skin conditions.

115. **Efficacy** - The ability of a drug to produce a desired or intended result in clinical settings.

600 QUESTION AND ANSWER

- What is the meaning of the prefix "brady-"?
  Answer: Slow - The prefix "brady-" is used in medical terminology to indicate slowness. For example, "bradycardia" refers to a slower than normal heart rate.

- What does the suffix "-ectomy" refer to?
  Answer: Surgical removal - The suffix "-ectomy" denotes the surgical removal of a specific part of the body. For instance, "appendectomy" is the surgical removal of the appendix.

- What is the root word in "gastroenterology"?
  Answer: Gastro - The root word "gastro" refers to the stomach. "Gastroenterology" is the study of the stomach and intestines.

- What does the prefix "hyper-" mean?
  Answer: Excessive or above normal - The prefix "hyper-" indicates an excessive amount or above normal. For example, "hypertension" means high blood pressure.

- What does the suffix "-itis" indicate?
  Answer: Inflammation - The suffix "-itis" is used to denote inflammation. For example, "arthritis" refers to inflammation of the joints.

- What does the term "cardiomegaly" mean?
  Answer: Enlarged heart - "Cardiomegaly" is a term used to describe an enlarged heart, with "cardio" referring to the heart and "megaly" indicating enlargement.

- What is the meaning of the prefix "tachy-"?
  Answer: Fast - The prefix "tachy-" is used to indicate rapidity or speed. For example, "tachycardia" refers to a fast heart rate.

- What does the suffix "-logy" mean?
  Answer: Study of - The suffix "-logy" denotes the study of a particular subject. For example, "neurology" is the study of the nervous system.

- What does the root word "nephro" refer to?
  Answer: Kidney - The root word "nephro" pertains to the kidney. For example, "nephrology" is the study of kidney function and diseases.

- What does the prefix "hypo-" mean?
  Answer: Below normal or deficient - The prefix "hypo-" indicates a deficiency or below normal levels. For example, "hypoglycemia" means low blood sugar levels.

- What does the suffix "-oma" indicate?
  Answer: Tumor or mass - The suffix "-oma" is used to denote a tumor or mass. For example, "carcinoma" refers to a type of cancerous tumor.

- What does the term "hepatomegaly" mean?
  Answer: Enlarged liver - "Hepatomegaly" refers to an enlarged liver, with "hepato" indicating the liver and "megaly" meaning enlargement.

- What is the meaning of the prefix "poly-"?
  Answer: Many or multiple - The prefix "poly-" indicates many or multiple. For example, "polyuria" means excessive urination.

- What does the suffix "-scopy" refer to?
  Answer: Visual examination - The suffix "-scopy" denotes a visual examination using a scope. For example, "endoscopy" is a procedure to visually examine the interior of a body organ.

- What does the root word "derm" refer to?
  Answer: Skin - The root word "derm" pertains to the skin. For example, "dermatology" is the study of skin conditions.

- What does the prefix "peri-" mean?
  Answer: Around or surrounding - The prefix "peri-" indicates around or surrounding. For example, "pericardium" refers to the membrane surrounding the heart.

- What does the suffix "-graphy" mean?
  Answer: Process of recording - The suffix "-graphy" denotes the process of recording or imaging. For example, "angiography" is the imaging of blood vessels.

- What does the term "osteoporosis" mean?
  Answer: Condition of porous bones - "Osteoporosis" refers to a condition where bones become porous and fragile, with "osteo" indicating bone and "porosis" meaning porous.

- What is the meaning of the prefix "auto-"?
  Answer: Self - The prefix "auto-" indicates self. For example, "autoimmune" refers to the immune response against the body's own cells.

- What does the suffix "-plasty" refer to?
  Answer: Surgical repair - The suffix "-plasty" denotes surgical repair. For example, "rhinoplasty" is the surgical repair of the nose.

- What does the root word "myo" refer to?
  Answer: Muscle - The root word "myo" pertains to muscle. For example, "myopathy" refers to a disease of the muscle.

- What does the prefix "endo-" mean?
  Answer: Within or inside - The prefix "endo-" indicates within or inside. For example, "endocrine" refers to glands that secrete hormones directly into the bloodstream.

- What does the suffix "-lysis" mean?
  Answer: Breakdown or destruction - The suffix "-lysis" denotes the breakdown or destruction of cells or substances. For example, "hemolysis" refers to the destruction of red blood cells.

- What does the root word "neuro" refer to?
  Answer: Nerve - The root word "neuro" pertains to nerves. For example, "neurology" is the study of the nervous system.

- What does the prefix "inter-" mean?
  Answer: Between - The prefix "inter-" indicates between. For example, "intercostal" refers to the space between the ribs.

- What does the suffix "-stomy" refer to?
  Answer: Creating an opening - The suffix "-stomy" denotes the creation of an opening. For example, "colostomy" is the surgical creation of an opening in the colon.

- What does the term "cyanosis" mean?
  Answer: Bluish discoloration of the skin - "Cyanosis" refers to a bluish discoloration of the skin due to lack of oxygen, with "cyano" indicating blue.

- What is the meaning of the prefix "trans-"?
  Answer: Across or through - The prefix "trans-" indicates across or through. For example, "transdermal" refers to something that goes through the skin.

- What does the suffix "-phobia" mean?
  Answer: Fear - The suffix "-phobia" denotes an irrational fear. For example, "arachnophobia" is the fear of spiders.

- What does the root word "hemo" refer to?
  Answer: Blood - The root word "hemo" pertains to blood. For example, "hemoglobin" is the protein in red blood cells that carries oxygen.

- What does the prefix "sub-" mean?
  Answer: Under or below - The prefix "sub-" indicates under or below. For example, "subcutaneous" refers to something situated or applied under the skin.

- What does the suffix "-algia" mean?
  Answer: Pain - The suffix "-algia" denotes pain. For example, "neuralgia" refers to nerve pain.

- What does the term "leukopenia" mean?
  Answer: Low white blood cell count - "Leukopenia" refers to a decrease in the number of white blood cells, with "leuko" indicating white and "penia" meaning deficiency.

- What is the meaning of the prefix "epi-"?
  Answer: Upon or above - The prefix "epi-" indicates upon or above. For example, "epidermis" refers to the outer layer of skin.

- What does the suffix "-rrhea" mean?
  Answer: Flow or discharge - The suffix "-rrhea" denotes flow or discharge. For example, "diarrhea" refers to the frequent discharge of liquid stool.

- What does the root word "arthro" refer to?
  Answer: Joint - The root word "arthro" pertains to joints. For example, "arthritis" is the inflammation of joints.

- What does the prefix "retro-" mean?
  Answer: Backward or behind - The prefix "retro-" indicates backward or behind. For example, "retroperitoneal" refers to the area behind the peritoneum.

- What does the suffix "-cyte" mean?
  Answer: Cell - The suffix "-cyte" denotes a cell. For example, "erythrocyte" refers to a red blood cell.

- What does the term "tachypnea" mean?
  Answer: Rapid breathing - "Tachypnea" refers to abnormally rapid breathing, with "tachy" indicating fast and "pnea" meaning breathing.

- What is the meaning of the prefix "anti-"?
  Answer: Against - The prefix "anti-" indicates against. For example, "antibiotic" refers to a substance that works against bacteria.

- What does the suffix "-genesis" mean?
  Answer: Formation or production - The suffix "-genesis" denotes formation or production. For example, "osteogenesis" refers to the formation of bone.

- What does the root word "cardio" refer to?
  Answer: Heart - The root word "cardio" pertains to the heart. For example, "cardiology" is the study of the heart and its functions.

- What does the prefix "intra-" mean?
  Answer: Within - The prefix "intra-" indicates within. For example, "intravenous" refers to something administered within a vein.

- What does the term "bradycardia" mean?
  Answer: Slow heart rate - "Bradycardia" refers to an abnormally slow heart rate, with "brady" indicating slow and "cardia" referring to the heart.

- What is the meaning of the prefix "peri-"?
  Answer: Around - The prefix "peri-" indicates around. For example, "pericardium" refers to the membrane surrounding the heart.

- What does the suffix "-ectomy" mean?
  Answer: Surgical removal - The suffix "-ectomy" denotes the surgical removal of a part of the body. For example, "appendectomy" is the surgical removal of the appendix.

- What does the root word "derm" refer to?
  Answer: Skin - The root word "derm" pertains to the skin. For example, "dermatology" is the study of skin and its diseases.

- What does the prefix "hypo-" mean?
  Answer: Under or below normal - The prefix "hypo-" indicates under or below normal. For example, "hypoglycemia" refers to low blood sugar levels.

- What does the suffix "-itis" mean?
  Answer: Inflammation - The suffix "-itis" denotes inflammation. For example, "tonsillitis" refers to the inflammation of the tonsils.

- What does the term "hyperthermia" mean?
  Answer: High body temperature - "Hyperthermia" refers to an abnormally high body temperature, with "hyper" indicating above normal and "thermia" referring to heat.

- What is the meaning of the prefix "poly-"?
  Answer: Many - The prefix "poly-" indicates many. For example, "polyuria" refers to the production of abnormally large volumes of urine.

- What does the suffix "-oma" mean?
  Answer: Tumor or mass - The suffix "-oma" denotes a tumor or mass. For example, "carcinoma" refers to a type of cancerous tumor.

- What does the root word "oste" refer to?
  Answer: Bone - The root word "oste" pertains to bones. For example, "osteoporosis" is a condition characterized by weakened bones.

- What does the prefix "pre-" mean?
  Answer: Before - The prefix "pre-" indicates before. For example, "prenatal" refers to the period before birth.

- What does the suffix "-plasty" mean?
  Answer: Surgical repair - The suffix "-plasty" denotes surgical repair. For example, "rhinoplasty" is the surgical repair or reshaping of the nose.

- What does the term "hemiplegia" mean?
  Answer: Paralysis of one side of the body - "Hemiplegia" refers to paralysis affecting one side of the body, with "hemi" indicating half and "plegia" meaning paralysis.

- What is the meaning of the prefix "post-"?
  Answer: After - The prefix "post-" indicates after. For example, "postoperative" refers to the period after surgery.

- What does the suffix "-scopy" mean?
  Answer: Visual examination - The suffix "-scopy" denotes a visual examination. For example, "endoscopy" is a procedure that allows doctors to view the inside of the body.

- What does the root word "hepato" refer to?
  Answer: Liver - The root word "hepato" pertains to the liver. For example, "hepatitis" is the inflammation of the liver.

- What does the prefix "auto-" mean?
  Answer: Self - The prefix "auto-" indicates self. For example, "autoimmune" refers to a condition where the immune system attacks the body's own tissues.

- What does the suffix "-graphy" mean?
  Answer: Process of recording - The suffix "-graphy" denotes the process of recording. For example, "angiography" is the imaging of blood vessels.

- What does the term "dysphagia" mean?
  Answer: Difficulty swallowing - "Dysphagia" refers to difficulty swallowing, with "dys" indicating difficulty and "phagia" meaning swallowing.

- What is the meaning of the prefix "contra-"?
  Answer: Against or opposite - The prefix "contra-" indicates against or opposite. For example, "contraceptive" refers to a method or device that prevents pregnancy.

- What does the suffix "-emia" mean?
  Answer: Blood condition - The suffix "-emia" denotes a blood condition. For example, "anemia" refers to a condition characterized by a deficiency of red blood cells.

- What does the root word "myo" refer to?
  Answer: Muscle - The root word "myo" pertains to muscles. For example, "myopathy" is a disease affecting muscle tissue.

- What does the suffix "-lysis" mean?
  Answer: Breakdown or destruction - The suffix "-lysis" denotes the breakdown or destruction of a substance. For example, "hemolysis" refers to the destruction of red blood cells.

- What does the term "tachycardia" mean?
  Answer: Fast heart rate - "Tachycardia" refers to an abnormally fast heart rate, with "tachy" indicating fast and "cardia" referring to the heart.

- What is the meaning of the prefix "trans-"?
  Answer: Across or through - The prefix "trans-" indicates across or through. For example, "transdermal" refers to the delivery of medication through the skin.

- What does the suffix "-stomy" mean?
  Answer: Creation of an opening - The suffix "-stomy" denotes the creation of an opening. For example, "colostomy" is a surgical procedure that creates an opening in the colon.

- What does the root word "nephro" refer to?
  Answer: Kidney - The root word "nephro" pertains to the kidneys. For example, "nephrology" is the study of kidney function and diseases.

- What does the prefix "epi-" mean?
  Answer: Upon or above - The prefix "epi-" indicates upon or above. For example, "epidermis" refers to the outer layer of skin.

- What does the suffix "-phobia" mean?
  Answer: Fear - The suffix "-phobia" denotes an irrational fear. For example, "arachnophobia" is the fear of spiders.

- What does the term "cyanosis" mean?
  Answer: Bluish discoloration of the skin - "Cyanosis" refers to a bluish discoloration of the skin due to lack of oxygen, with "cyan" indicating blue.

- What is the meaning of the prefix "inter-"?
  Answer: Between - The prefix "inter-" indicates between. For example, "intercostal" refers to the muscles located between the ribs.

- What does the suffix "-rrhea" mean?
  Answer: Flow or discharge - The suffix "-rrhea" denotes flow or discharge. For example, "diarrhea" refers to the frequent discharge of liquid stool.

- What does the root word "encephalo" refer to?
  Answer: Brain - The root word "encephalo" pertains to the brain. For example, "encephalitis" is the inflammation of the brain.

- What does the prefix "retro-" mean?
  Answer: Backward or behind - The prefix "retro-" indicates backward or behind. For example, "retrograde" refers to moving backward.

- What does the suffix "-tomy" mean?
  Answer: Cutting or incision - The suffix "-tomy" denotes cutting or making an incision. For example, "tracheotomy" is a surgical procedure that involves making an incision in the trachea.

- What does the term "leukopenia" mean?
  Answer: Low white blood cell count - "Leukopenia" refers to a low white blood cell count, with "leuko" indicating white and "penia" meaning deficiency.

- What is the meaning of the prefix "sub-"?
  Answer: Under or below - The prefix "sub-" indicates under or below. For example, "subcutaneous" refers to something located under the skin.

- What does the suffix "-algia" mean?
  Answer: Pain - The suffix "-algia" denotes pain. For example, "neuralgia" refers to nerve pain.

- What does the root word "thoraco" refer to?
  Answer: Chest - The root word "thoraco" pertains to the chest. For example, "thoracotomy" is a surgical procedure involving an incision into the chest wall.

- What does the prefix "bi-" mean?
  Answer: Two - The prefix "bi-" indicates two. For example, "bicuspid" refers to a structure with two cusps or points.

- What does the suffix "-megaly" mean?
  Answer: Enlargement - The suffix "-megaly" denotes enlargement. For example, "cardiomegaly" refers to the enlargement of the heart.

- What does the term "hypoxia" mean?
  Answer: Low oxygen levels - "Hypoxia" refers to low oxygen levels in the tissues, with "hypo" indicating below normal and "oxia" referring to oxygen.

- What is the meaning of the prefix "tri-"?
  Answer: Three - The prefix "tri-" indicates three. For example, "triceps" refers to a muscle with three heads or points of origin.

- What does the root word "dermato" refer to?
  Answer: Skin - The root word "dermato" pertains to the skin. For example, "dermatology" is the branch of medicine dealing with skin conditions.

- What does the prefix "peri-" mean?
  Answer: Around - The prefix "peri-" indicates around. For example, "pericardium" refers to the membrane surrounding the heart.

- What does the suffix "-emia" mean?
  Answer: Blood condition - The suffix "-emia" denotes a blood condition. For example, "anemia" refers to a condition characterized by a deficiency of red blood cells.

- What does the term "bradycardia" mean?
  Answer: Slow heart rate - "Bradycardia" refers to an abnormally slow heart rate, with "brady" indicating slow and "cardia" referring to the heart.

- What is the meaning of the prefix "hyper-"?
  Answer: Excessive or above normal - The prefix "hyper-" indicates excessive or above normal. For example, "hypertension" refers to abnormally high blood pressure.

- What does the suffix "-plasty" mean?
  Answer: Surgical repair - The suffix "-plasty" denotes surgical repair. For example, "rhinoplasty" is a surgical procedure to repair or reshape the nose.

- What does the root word "osteo" refer to?
  Answer: Bone - The root word "osteo" pertains to bones. For example, "osteoporosis" is a condition characterized by weakened bones.

- What does the prefix "intra-" mean?
  Answer: Within - The prefix "intra-" indicates within. For example, "intravenous" refers to something administered within a vein.

- What does the suffix "-itis" mean?
  Answer: Inflammation - The suffix "-itis" denotes inflammation. For example, "arthritis" refers to inflammation of the joints.

- What does the term "hematuria" mean?
  Answer: Blood in the urine - "Hematuria" refers to the presence of blood in the urine, with "hema" indicating blood and "uria" referring to urine.

- What is the meaning of the prefix "poly-"?
  Answer: Many - The prefix "poly-" indicates many. For example, "polyuria" refers to the production of abnormally large volumes of urine.

- What does the suffix "-oma" mean?
  Answer: Tumor or mass - The suffix "-oma" denotes a tumor or mass. For example, "carcinoma" refers to a type of cancerous tumor.

- What does the root word "hepato" refer to?
  Answer: Liver - The root word "hepato" pertains to the liver. For example, "hepatitis" is the inflammation of the liver.

- What does the prefix "ante-" mean?
  Answer: Before - The prefix "ante-" indicates before. For example, "antenatal" refers to the period before birth.

- What does the suffix "-lysis" mean?
  Answer: Breakdown or destruction - The suffix "-lysis" denotes the breakdown or destruction of a substance. For example, "hemolysis" refers to the destruction of red blood cells.

- What does the term "tachycardia" mean?
  Answer: Fast heart rate - "Tachycardia" refers to an abnormally fast heart rate, with "tachy" indicating fast and "cardia" referring to the heart.

- What is the meaning of the prefix "trans-"?
  Answer: Across or through - The prefix "trans-" indicates across or through. For example, "transdermal" refers to the delivery of medication through the skin.

- What does the suffix "-stomy" mean?
  Answer: Creation of an opening - The suffix "-stomy" denotes the creation of an opening. For example, "colostomy" is a surgical procedure that creates an opening in the colon.

- What does the root word "nephro" refer to?
  Answer: Kidney - The root word "nephro" pertains to the kidneys. For example, "nephrology" is the study of kidney function and diseases.

- What does the prefix "epi-" mean?
  Answer: Upon or above - The prefix "epi-" indicates upon or above. For example, "epidermis" refers to the outer layer of skin.

- What does the suffix "-phobia" mean?
  Answer: Fear - The suffix "-phobia" denotes an irrational fear. For example, "arachnophobia" is the fear of spiders.

- What is the meaning of the prefix "retro-"?
  Answer: Backward or behind - The prefix "retro-" indicates backward or behind. For example, "retroperitoneal" refers to the anatomical space behind the peritoneum.

- What does the suffix "-ectomy" mean?
  Answer: Surgical removal - The suffix "-ectomy" denotes the surgical removal of a part of the body. For example, "appendectomy" is the surgical removal of the appendix.

- What does the root word "cardio" refer to?
  Answer: Heart - The root word "cardio" pertains to the heart. For example, "cardiology" is the study of heart diseases and conditions.

- What does the prefix "hypo-" mean?
  Answer: Below normal or deficient - The prefix "hypo-" indicates below normal or deficient. For example, "hypoglycemia" refers to abnormally low blood sugar levels.

- What does the suffix "-graphy" mean?
  Answer: Process of recording or imaging - The suffix "-graphy" denotes the process of recording or imaging. For example, "angiography" is the imaging of blood vessels.

- What does the term "leukopenia" mean?
  Answer: Low white blood cell count - "Leukopenia" refers to a decrease in the number of white blood cells, with "leuko" indicating white and "penia" indicating deficiency.

- What is the meaning of the prefix "inter-"?
  Answer: Between - The prefix "inter-" indicates between. For example, "intercostal" refers to the space between the ribs.

- What does the suffix "-logy" mean?
  Answer: Study of - The suffix "-logy" denotes the study of a particular subject. For example, "neurology" is the study of the nervous system.

- What does the root word "myo" refer to?
  Answer: Muscle - The root word "myo" pertains to muscles. For example, "myopathy" refers to a disease of the muscle tissue.

- What does the prefix "sub-" mean?
  Answer: Under or below - The prefix "sub-" indicates under or below. For example, "subcutaneous" refers to something situated or applied under the skin.

- What does the suffix "-scopy" mean?
  Answer: Visual examination - The suffix "-scopy" denotes a visual examination. For example, "endoscopy" is a procedure that allows doctors to view the inside of the body.

- What does the term "hyperglycemia" mean?
  Answer: High blood sugar - "Hyperglycemia" refers to abnormally high blood sugar levels, with "hyper" indicating excessive and "glycemia" referring to sugar in the blood.

- What is the meaning of the prefix "post-"?
  Answer: After - The prefix "post-" indicates after. For example, "postoperative" refers to the period after surgery.

- What does the suffix "-pathy" mean?
  Answer: Disease or disorder - The suffix "-pathy" denotes a disease or disorder. For example, "neuropathy" refers to a disease affecting the nerves.

- What does the root word "pulmo" refer to?
  Answer: Lung - The root word "pulmo" pertains to the lungs. For example, "pulmonology" is the study of lung diseases and conditions.

- What does the prefix "anti-" mean?
  Answer: Against - The prefix "anti-" indicates against. For example, "antibiotic" refers to a substance that works against bacteria.

- What does the suffix "-rrhea" mean?
  Answer: Flow or discharge - The suffix "-rrhea" denotes flow or discharge. For example, "diarrhea" refers to the frequent discharge of liquid stool.

- What does the term "osteoporosis" mean?
  Answer: Weakening of bones - "Osteoporosis" refers to a condition characterized by weakened bones, with "osteo" indicating bone and "porosis" indicating porous or weak.

- What is the meaning of the prefix "pre-"?
  Answer: Before - The prefix "pre-" indicates before. For example, "prenatal" refers to the period before birth.

- What does the suffix "-tomy" mean?
  Answer: Cutting or incision - The suffix "-tomy" denotes cutting or making an incision. For example, "tracheotomy" is a surgical procedure to create an opening in the trachea.

- What does the root word "neuro" refer to?
  Answer: Nerve - The root word "neuro" pertains to nerves. For example, "neurology" is the study of the nervous system.

- What does the suffix "-lysis" mean?
  Answer: Breakdown or destruction - The suffix "-lysis" denotes the breakdown or destruction of cells or substances. For example, "hemolysis" refers to the destruction of red blood cells.

- What does the term "tachycardia" mean?
  Answer: Fast heart rate - "Tachycardia" refers to an abnormally fast heart rate, with "tachy" indicating rapid and "cardia" referring to the heart.

- What is the meaning of the prefix "trans-"?
  Answer: Across or through - The prefix "trans-" indicates across or through. For example, "transdermal" refers to something administered across the skin.

- What does the suffix "-stasis" mean?
  Answer: Stopping or controlling - The suffix "-stasis" denotes stopping or controlling. For example, "hemostasis" refers to the stopping of bleeding.

- What does the root word "derm" refer to?
  Answer: Skin - The root word "derm" pertains to the skin. For example, "dermatology" is the study of skin diseases and conditions.

- What does the prefix "epi-" mean?
  Answer: Upon or above - The prefix "epi-" indicates upon or above. For example, "epidermis" refers to the outer layer of skin.

- What does the suffix "-phobia" mean?
  Answer: Fear - The suffix "-phobia" denotes an irrational fear. For example, "arachnophobia" is the fear of spiders.

- What does the term "bradycardia" mean?
  Answer: Slow heart rate - "Bradycardia" refers to an abnormally slow heart rate, with "brady" indicating slow and "cardia" referring to the heart.

- What is the meaning of the prefix "poly-"?
  Answer: Many or much - The prefix "poly-" indicates many or much. For example, "polyuria" refers to the production of abnormally large volumes of urine.

- What does the suffix "-algia" mean?
  Answer: Pain - The suffix "-algia" denotes pain. For example, "neuralgia" refers to nerve pain.

- What does the root word "hepat" refer to?
  Answer: Liver - The root word "hepat" pertains to the liver. For example, "hepatitis" is the inflammation of the liver.

- What does the prefix "auto-" mean?
  Answer: Self - The prefix "auto-" indicates self. For example, "autoimmune" refers to a condition where the immune system attacks the body's own cells.

- What does the suffix "-emia" mean?
  Answer: Blood condition - The suffix "-emia" denotes a blood condition. For example, "anemia" refers to a deficiency of red blood cells or hemoglobin.

- What does the term "nephrology" mean?
  Answer: Study of the kidneys - "Nephrology" refers to the study of kidney diseases and conditions, with "nephro" indicating kidney and "logy" indicating the study of.

- What is the meaning of the prefix "pseudo-"?
  Answer: False - The prefix "pseudo-" indicates false. For example, "pseudocyst" refers to a false cyst that lacks an epithelial lining.

- What does the suffix "-itis" mean?
  Answer: Inflammation - The suffix "-itis" denotes inflammation. For example, "arthritis" refers to the inflammation of the joints.

- What does the root word "gastr" refer to?
  Answer: Stomach - The root word "gastr" pertains to the stomach. For example, "gastritis" is the inflammation of the stomach lining.

- What does the prefix "bi-" mean?
  Answer: Two - The prefix "bi-" indicates two. For example, "bicuspid" refers to a structure with two cusps or points.

- What does the suffix "-oma" mean?
  Answer: Tumor or mass - The suffix "-oma" denotes a tumor or mass. For example, "carcinoma" refers to a type of cancerous tumor.

- What does the term "hypotension" mean?
  Answer: Low blood pressure - "Hypotension" refers to abnormally low blood pressure, with "hypo" indicating below normal and "tension" referring to pressure.

- What is the meaning of the prefix "tri-"?
  Answer: Three - The prefix "tri-" indicates three. For example, "tricuspid" refers to a structure with three cusps or points.

- What does the suffix "-plasty" mean?
  Answer: Surgical repair - The suffix "-plasty" denotes surgical repair. For example, "rhinoplasty" is the surgical repair or reshaping of the nose.

- What is the meaning of the prefix "hyper-"?
  Answer: Excessive or above normal - The prefix "hyper-" indicates excessive or above normal. For example, "hyperglycemia" refers to an abnormally high level of glucose in the blood.

- What does the suffix "-ectomy" mean?
  Answer: Surgical removal - The suffix "-ectomy" denotes surgical removal. For example, "appendectomy" is the surgical removal of the appendix.

- What does the root word "oste" refer to?
  Answer: Bone - The root word "oste" pertains to bone. For example, "osteoporosis" is a condition characterized by weakened bones.

- What does the prefix "peri-" mean?
  Answer: Around - The prefix "peri-" indicates around. For example, "pericardium" refers to the membrane surrounding the heart.

- What does the suffix "-lysis" mean?
  Answer: Breakdown or destruction - The suffix "-lysis" denotes the breakdown or destruction of cells or substances. For example, "hemolysis" refers to the destruction of red blood cells.

- What does the term "tachycardia" mean?
  Answer: Fast heart rate - "Tachycardia" refers to an abnormally fast heart rate, with "tachy" indicating rapid and "cardia" referring to the heart.

- What is the meaning of the prefix "trans-"?
  Answer: Across or through - The prefix "trans-" indicates across or through. For example, "transdermal" refers to something administered across the skin.

- What does the suffix "-stasis" mean?
  Answer: Stopping or controlling - The suffix "-stasis" denotes stopping or controlling. For example, "hemostasis" refers to the stopping of bleeding.

- What does the root word "derm" refer to?
  Answer: Skin - The root word "derm" pertains to the skin. For example, "dermatology" is the study of skin diseases and conditions.

- What does the prefix "epi-" mean?
  Answer: Upon or above - The prefix "epi-" indicates upon or above. For example, "epidermis" refers to the outer layer of skin.

- What does the suffix "-phobia" mean?
  Answer: Fear - The suffix "-phobia" denotes an irrational fear. For example, "arachnophobia" is the fear of spiders.

- What does the term "bradycardia" mean?
  Answer: Slow heart rate - "Bradycardia" refers to an abnormally slow heart rate, with "brady" indicating slow and "cardia" referring to the heart.

- What is the meaning of the prefix "poly-"?
  Answer: Many or much - The prefix "poly-" indicates many or much. For example, "polyuria" refers to the production of abnormally large volumes of urine.

- What does the suffix "-algia" mean?
  Answer: Pain - The suffix "-algia" denotes pain. For example, "neuralgia" refers to nerve pain.

- What does the root word "hepat" refer to?
  Answer: Liver - The root word "hepat" pertains to the liver. For example, "hepatitis" is the inflammation of the liver.

- What does the prefix "auto-" mean?
  Answer: Self - The prefix "auto-" indicates self. For example, "autoimmune" refers to a condition where the immune system attacks the body's own cells.

- What does the suffix "-emia" mean?
  Answer: Blood condition - The suffix "-emia" denotes a blood condition. For example, "anemia" refers to a deficiency of red blood cells or hemoglobin.

- What does the term "nephrology" mean?
  Answer: Study of the kidneys - "Nephrology" refers to the study of kidney diseases and conditions, with "nephro" indicating kidney and "logy" indicating the study of.

- What is the meaning of the prefix "pseudo-"?
  Answer: False - The prefix "pseudo-" indicates false. For example, "pseudocyst" refers to a false cyst that lacks an epithelial lining.

- What does the suffix "-itis" mean?
  Answer: Inflammation - The suffix "-itis" denotes inflammation. For example, "arthritis" refers to the inflammation of the joints.

- What does the root word "gastr" refer to?
  Answer: Stomach - The root word "gastr" pertains to the stomach. For example, "gastritis" is the inflammation of the stomach lining.

- What does the suffix "-plasty" mean?
  Answer: Surgical repair - The suffix "-plasty" denotes surgical repair or reconstruction. For example, "rhinoplasty" is the surgical repair or reshaping of the nose.

- What does the root word "cardi" refer to?
  Answer: Heart - The root word "cardi" pertains to the heart. For example, "cardiology" is the study of heart diseases and conditions.

- What does the prefix "hypo-" mean?
  Answer: Below normal or deficient - The prefix "hypo-" indicates below normal or deficient. For example, "hypoglycemia" refers to abnormally low levels of glucose in the blood.

- What does the suffix "-oma" mean?
  Answer: Tumor or mass - The suffix "-oma" denotes a tumor or mass. For example, "carcinoma" refers to a type of cancerous tumor.

- What does the term "neurology" mean?
  Answer: Study of the nervous system - "Neurology" refers to the study of the nervous system and its disorders, with "neuro" indicating nerve and "logy" indicating the study of.

- What is the meaning of the prefix "inter-"?
  Answer: Between - The prefix "inter-" indicates between. For example, "intercostal" refers to something situated between the ribs.

- What does the suffix "-graphy" mean?
  Answer: Process of recording - The suffix "-graphy" denotes the process of recording or imaging. For example, "angiography" is the imaging of blood vessels.

- What does the root word "pulmon" refer to?
  Answer: Lung - The root word "pulmon" pertains to the lung. For example, "pulmonology" is the study of lung diseases and conditions.

- What does the prefix "retro-" mean?
  Answer: Backward or behind - The prefix "retro-" indicates backward or behind. For example, "retroperitoneal" refers to something located behind the peritoneum.

- What does the suffix "-scopy" mean?
  Answer: Visual examination - The suffix "-scopy" denotes visual examination. For example, "endoscopy" is the visual examination of the interior of a body organ or cavity.

- What does the term "dermatology" mean?
  Answer: Study of the skin - "Dermatology" refers to the study of skin diseases and conditions, with "derm" indicating skin and "logy" indicating the study of.

- What is the meaning of the prefix "sub-"?
  Answer: Under or below - The prefix "sub-" indicates under or below. For example, "subcutaneous" refers to something situated or applied under the skin.

- What does the suffix "-megaly" mean?
  Answer: Enlargement - The suffix "-megaly" denotes enlargement. For example, "hepatomegaly" refers to the enlargement of the liver.

- What does the root word "nephr" refer to?
  Answer: Kidney - The root word "nephr" pertains to the kidney. For example, "nephritis" is the inflammation of the kidneys.

- What does the prefix "anti-" mean?
  Answer: Against - The prefix "anti-" indicates against. For example, "antibiotic" refers to a substance that works against bacteria.

- What does the suffix "-pathy" mean?
  Answer: Disease or disorder - The suffix "-pathy" denotes disease or disorder. For example, "neuropathy" refers to a disease or disorder of the nerves.

- What does the term "oncology" mean?
  Answer: Study of tumors - "Oncology" refers to the study of tumors and cancer, with "onco" indicating tumor and "logy" indicating the study of.

- What is the meaning of the prefix "peri-"?
  Answer: Around - The prefix "peri-" indicates around. For example, "pericardium" refers to the membrane surrounding the heart.

- What does the suffix "-rrhea" mean?
  Answer: Flow or discharge - The suffix "-rrhea" denotes flow or discharge. For example, "diarrhea" refers to the frequent flow of loose or watery stools.

- What does the root word "arthr" refer to?
  Answer: Joint - The root word "arthr" pertains to joints. For example, "arthritis" is the inflammation of the joints.

- What does the prefix "endo-" mean?
  Answer: Within or inside - The prefix "endo-" indicates within or inside. For example, "endoscopy" refers to the visual examination of the interior of a body organ or cavity.

- What does the root word "hepat" refer to?
  Answer: Liver - The root word "hepat" pertains to the liver. For example, "hepatitis" is the inflammation of the liver.

- What does the prefix "tachy-" mean?
  Answer: Fast or rapid - The prefix "tachy-" indicates fast or rapid. For example, "tachycardia" refers to an abnormally fast heart rate.

- What does the suffix "-lysis" mean?
  Answer: Breakdown or destruction - The suffix "-lysis" denotes breakdown or destruction. For example, "hemolysis" refers to the destruction of red blood cells.

- What does the root word "gastr" refer to?
  Answer: Stomach - The root word "gastr" pertains to the stomach. For example, "gastritis" is the inflammation of the stomach lining.

- What does the prefix "brady-" mean?
  Answer: Slow - The prefix "brady-" indicates slow. For example, "bradycardia" refers to an abnormally slow heart rate.

- What does the suffix "-stomy" mean?
  Answer: Creating an opening - The suffix "-stomy" denotes creating an opening. For example, "colostomy" refers to the surgical creation of an opening from the colon to the outside of the body.

- What does the root word "myo" refer to?
  Answer: Muscle - The root word "myo" pertains to muscle. For example, "myopathy" refers to a disease of the muscle.

- What does the prefix "hyper-" mean?
  Answer: Above normal or excessive - The prefix "hyper-" indicates above normal or excessive. For example, "hypertension" refers to abnormally high blood pressure.

- What does the suffix "-emia" mean?
  Answer: Blood condition - The suffix "-emia" denotes a blood condition. For example, "anemia" refers to a condition characterized by a deficiency of red blood cells or hemoglobin.

- What does the root word "oste" refer to?
  Answer: Bone - The root word "oste" pertains to bone. For example, "osteoporosis" is a condition characterized by weakened bones.

- What does the prefix "poly-" mean?
  Answer: Many or multiple - The prefix "poly-" indicates many or multiple. For example, "polyuria" refers to the production of abnormally large volumes of urine.

- What does the suffix "-itis" mean?
  Answer: Inflammation - The suffix "-itis" denotes inflammation. For example, "appendicitis" is the inflammation of the appendix.

- What does the root word "derm" refer to?
  Answer: Skin - The root word "derm" pertains to the skin. For example, "dermatitis" is the inflammation of the skin.

- What does the prefix "peri-" mean?
  Answer: Around - The prefix "peri-" indicates around. For example, "pericarditis" refers to the inflammation of the pericardium, the membrane surrounding the heart.

- What does the suffix "-ectomy" mean?
  Answer: Surgical removal - The suffix "-ectomy" denotes surgical removal. For example, "appendectomy" refers to the surgical removal of the appendix.

- What does the root word "neuro" refer to?
  Answer: Nerve - The root word "neuro" pertains to nerves. For example, "neurology" is the study of the nervous system and its disorders.

- What does the prefix "trans-" mean?
  Answer: Across or through - The prefix "trans-" indicates across or through. For example, "transdermal" refers to something administered across the skin.

- What does the suffix "-algia" mean?
  Answer: Pain - The suffix "-algia" denotes pain. For example, "neuralgia" refers to nerve pain.

- What does the root word "cyt" refer to?
  Answer: Cell - The root word "cyt" pertains to cells. For example, "cytology" is the study of cells.

- What does the prefix "intra-" mean?
  Answer: Within or inside - The prefix "intra-" indicates within or inside. For example, "intravenous" refers to something administered within a vein.

- What does the suffix "-genesis" mean?
  Answer: Formation or origin - The suffix "-genesis" denotes formation or origin. For example, "osteogenesis" refers to the formation of bone.

- What does the root word "hemat" refer to?
  Answer: Blood - The root word "hemat" pertains to blood. For example, "hematology" is the study of blood and its disorders.

- What does the suffix "-phobia" mean?
  Answer: Fear - The suffix "-phobia" denotes fear. For example, "arachnophobia" refers to an intense fear of spiders.

- What does the root word "cardi" refer to?
  Answer: Heart - The root word "cardi" pertains to the heart. For example, "cardiology" is the study of the heart and its functions.

- What does the prefix "endo-" mean?
  Answer: Within or inside - The prefix "endo-" indicates within or inside. For example, "endoscopy" refers to a procedure that looks inside the body using an instrument called an endoscope.

- What does the suffix "-pathy" mean?
  Answer: Disease or disorder - The suffix "-pathy" denotes disease or disorder. For example, "neuropathy" refers to a disease or dysfunction of one or more peripheral nerves.

- What does the root word "pulmon" refer to?
  Answer: Lung - The root word "pulmon" pertains to the lungs. For example, "pulmonology" is the study of lung diseases.

- What does the prefix "inter-" mean?
  Answer: Between - The prefix "inter-" indicates between. For example, "intercellular" refers to something occurring between cells.

- What does the suffix "-plasty" mean?
  Answer: Surgical repair - The suffix "-plasty" denotes surgical repair. For example, "rhinoplasty" refers to the surgical repair or reshaping of the nose.

- What does the root word "nephr" refer to?
  Answer: Kidney - The root word "nephr" pertains to the kidneys. For example, "nephrology" is the study of kidney function and diseases.

- What does the prefix "retro-" mean?
  Answer: Backward or behind - The prefix "retro-" indicates backward or behind. For example, "retroperitoneal" refers to the anatomical space in the abdominal cavity behind the peritoneum.

- What does the suffix "-rrhea" mean?
  Answer: Flow or discharge - The suffix "-rrhea" denotes flow or discharge. For example, "diarrhea" refers to the condition of having frequent and watery bowel movements.

- What does the root word "encephal" refer to?
  Answer: Brain - The root word "encephal" pertains to the brain. For example, "encephalitis" is the inflammation of the brain.

- What does the prefix "sub-" mean?
  Answer: Under or below - The prefix "sub-" indicates under or below. For example, "subcutaneous" refers to something situated or applied under the skin.

- What does the suffix "-oma" mean?
  Answer: Tumor or mass - The suffix "-oma" denotes a tumor or mass. For example, "carcinoma" refers to a type of cancer that begins in the skin or in tissues that line or cover internal organs.

- What does the root word "arthr" refer to?
  Answer: Joint - The root word "arthr" pertains to joints. For example, "arthritis" is the inflammation of one or more joints.

- What does the prefix "epi-" mean?
  Answer: Upon or above - The prefix "epi-" indicates upon or above. For example, "epidermis" refers to the outer layer of skin cells.

- What does the suffix "-scopy" mean?
  Answer: Visual examination - The suffix "-scopy" denotes visual examination. For example, "colonoscopy" refers to the visual examination of the colon using a colonoscope.

- What does the root word "glyc" refer to?
  Answer: Sugar or glucose - The root word "glyc" pertains to sugar or glucose. For example, "glycemia" refers to the presence of glucose in the blood.

- What does the prefix "contra-" mean?
  Answer: Against or opposite - The prefix "contra-" indicates against or opposite. For example, "contraceptive" refers to a method or device serving to prevent pregnancy.

- What does the suffix "-graphy" mean?
  Answer: Process of recording - The suffix "-graphy" denotes the process of recording. For example, "angiography" refers to the imaging of blood vessels.

- What does the root word "phleb" refer to?
  Answer: Vein - The root word "phleb" pertains to veins. For example, "phlebitis" is the inflammation of a vein.

- What does the suffix "-lysis" mean?
  Answer: Breakdown or destruction - The suffix "-lysis" denotes breakdown or destruction. For example, "hemolysis" refers to the destruction of red blood cells.

- What does the root word "derm" refer to?
  Answer: Skin - The root word "derm" pertains to the skin. For example, "dermatology" is the study of skin and its diseases.

- What does the prefix "peri-" mean?
  Answer: Around or surrounding - The prefix "peri-" indicates around or surrounding. For example, "pericardium" refers to the membrane enclosing the heart.

- What does the suffix "-stomy" mean?
  Answer: Creation of an opening - The suffix "-stomy" denotes the creation of an opening. For example, "colostomy" refers to a surgical procedure that creates an opening from the colon to the surface of the body.

- What does the root word "hepat" refer to?
  Answer: Liver - The root word "hepat" pertains to the liver. For example, "hepatitis" is the inflammation of the liver.

- What does the prefix "trans-" mean?
  Answer: Across or through - The prefix "trans-" indicates across or through. For example, "transdermal" refers to the administration of medication through the skin.

- What does the suffix "-emia" mean?
  Answer: Blood condition - The suffix "-emia" denotes a blood condition. For example, "anemia" refers to a condition in which there is a deficiency of red blood cells or hemoglobin in the blood.

- What does the root word "myo" refer to?
  Answer: Muscle - The root word "myo" pertains to muscles. For example, "myopathy" refers to a disease of muscle tissue.

- What does the prefix "hyper-" mean?
  Answer: Above normal or excessive - The prefix "hyper-" indicates above normal or excessive. For example, "hypertension" refers to abnormally high blood pressure.

- What does the suffix "-ectomy" mean?
  Answer: Surgical removal - The suffix "-ectomy" denotes surgical removal. For example, "appendectomy" refers to the surgical removal of the appendix.

- What does the root word "oste" refer to?
  Answer: Bone - The root word "oste" pertains to bones. For example, "osteoporosis" is a condition characterized by weakened bones.

- What does the prefix "intra-" mean?
  Answer: Within or inside - The prefix "intra-" indicates within or inside. For example, "intravenous" refers to something administered within or into a vein.

- What does the suffix "-itis" mean?
  Answer: Inflammation - The suffix "-itis" denotes inflammation. For example, "bronchitis" refers to the inflammation of the bronchial tubes.

- What does the root word "neur" refer to?
  Answer: Nerve - The root word "neur" pertains to nerves. For example, "neurology" is the study of the nervous system and its disorders.

- What does the prefix "pre-" mean?
  Answer: Before - The prefix "pre-" indicates before. For example, "prenatal" refers to the period before birth.

- What does the suffix "-logy" mean?
  Answer: Study of - The suffix "-logy" denotes the study of. For example, "biology" is the study of living organisms.

- What does the root word "gastr" refer to?
  Answer: Stomach - The root word "gastr" pertains to the stomach. For example, "gastritis" is the inflammation of the stomach lining.

- What does the prefix "post-" mean?
  Answer: After - The prefix "post-" indicates after. For example, "postoperative" refers to the period after surgery.

- What does the suffix "-megaly" mean?
  Answer: Enlargement - The suffix "-megaly" denotes enlargement. For example, "cardiomegaly" refers to the enlargement of the heart.

- What does the root word "hemat" refer to?
  Answer: Blood - The root word "hemat" pertains to blood. For example, "hematology" is the study of blood and its disorders.

- What does the prefix "anti-" mean?
  Answer: Against - The prefix "anti-" indicates against. For example, "antibiotic" refers to a substance that works against bacteria.

- What does the suffix "-oma" mean?
  Answer: Tumor or mass - The suffix "-oma" denotes a tumor or mass. For example, "melanoma" refers to a type of skin cancer that develops from the pigment-producing cells known as melanocytes.

- What does the prefix "sub-" mean?
  Answer: Under or below - The prefix "sub-" indicates under or below. For example, "subcutaneous" refers to something situated or applied under the skin.

- What does the suffix "-pathy" mean?
  Answer: Disease or disorder - The suffix "-pathy" denotes a disease or disorder. For example, "neuropathy" refers to a disease or dysfunction of one or more peripheral nerves.

- What does the root word "cardi" refer to?
  Answer: Heart - The root word "cardi" pertains to the heart. For example, "cardiology" is the study of the heart and its functions.

- What does the prefix "epi-" mean?
  Answer: Upon or above - The prefix "epi-" indicates upon or above. For example, "epidermis" refers to the outer layer of skin cells.

- What does the suffix "-plasty" mean?
  Answer: Surgical repair - The suffix "-plasty" denotes surgical repair. For example, "rhinoplasty" refers to the surgical repair or reshaping of the nose.

- What does the root word "pulmon" refer to?
  Answer: Lung - The root word "pulmon" pertains to the lungs. For example, "pulmonology" is the study of lung diseases.

- What does the prefix "brady-" mean?
  Answer: Slow - The prefix "brady-" indicates slow. For example, "bradycardia" refers to a slower than normal heart rate.

- What does the suffix "-rrhea" mean?
  Answer: Flow or discharge - The suffix "-rrhea" denotes flow or discharge. For example, "diarrhea" refers to the condition of having frequent and liquid bowel movements.

- What does the root word "arthr" refer to?
  Answer: Joint - The root word "arthr" pertains to joints. For example, "arthritis" is the inflammation of one or more joints.

- What does the prefix "tachy-" mean?
  Answer: Fast - The prefix "tachy-" indicates fast. For example, "tachycardia" refers to a faster than normal heart rate.

- What does the suffix "-scopy" mean?
  Answer: Visual examination - The suffix "-scopy" denotes visual examination. For example, "endoscopy" refers to a procedure that uses an instrument to view the inside of the body.

- What does the root word "cyt" refer to?
  Answer: Cell - The root word "cyt" pertains to cells. For example, "cytology" is the study of cells.

- What does the prefix "hypo-" mean?
  Answer: Below normal or deficient - The prefix "hypo-" indicates below normal or deficient. For example, "hypoglycemia" refers to abnormally low blood sugar levels.

- What does the suffix "-graphy" mean?
  Answer: Process of recording - The suffix "-graphy" denotes the process of recording. For example, "angiography" is the imaging of blood vessels.

- What does the root word "nephr" refer to?
  Answer: Kidney - The root word "nephr" pertains to the kidneys. For example, "nephrology" is the study of kidney function and diseases.

- What does the prefix "inter-" mean?
  Answer: Between - The prefix "inter-" indicates between. For example, "intercostal" refers to something situated between the ribs.

- What does the suffix "-lysis" mean?
  Answer: Breakdown or destruction - The suffix "-lysis" denotes breakdown or destruction. For example, "dialysis" refers to the process of removing waste products and excess fluid from the blood when the kidneys are not functioning properly.

- What does the root word "encephal" refer to?
  Answer: Brain - The root word "encephal" pertains to the brain. For example, "encephalopathy" refers to any disease of the brain.

- What does the prefix "retro-" mean?
  Answer: Backward or behind - The prefix "retro-" indicates backward or behind. For example, "retroperitoneal" refers to the anatomical space in the abdominal cavity behind the peritoneum.

- What does the suffix "-tomy" mean?
  Answer: Cutting or incision - The suffix "-tomy" denotes cutting or incision. For example, "tracheotomy" refers to a surgical procedure to create an opening in the trachea.

- What does the root word "glyc" refer to?
  Answer: Sugar - The root word "glyc" pertains to sugar. For example, "glycemia" refers to the presence of glucose in the blood.

- What does the suffix "-emia" mean?
  Answer: Blood condition - The suffix "-emia" denotes a blood condition. For example, "anemia" refers to a condition in which there is a deficiency of red blood cells or hemoglobin in the blood.

- What does the root word "derm" refer to?
  Answer: Skin - The root word "derm" pertains to the skin. For example, "dermatology" is the branch of medicine dealing with the skin and its diseases.

- What does the prefix "peri-" mean?
  Answer: Around - The prefix "peri-" indicates around. For example, "pericardium" refers to the membrane enclosing the heart.

- What does the suffix "-stasis" mean?
  Answer: Stopping or controlling - The suffix "-stasis" denotes stopping or controlling. For example, "hemostasis" refers to the process of stopping bleeding.

- What does the root word "hepat" refer to?
  Answer: Liver - The root word "hepat" pertains to the liver. For example, "hepatitis" is the inflammation of the liver.

- What does the prefix "poly-" mean?
  Answer: Many - The prefix "poly-" indicates many. For example, "polyuria" refers to the production of abnormally large volumes of dilute urine.

- What does the suffix "-phobia" mean?
  Answer: Fear - The suffix "-phobia" denotes fear. For example, "claustrophobia" refers to the fear of confined spaces.

- What does the root word "oste" refer to?
  Answer: Bone - The root word "oste" pertains to bones. For example, "osteoporosis" is a condition characterized by weak and brittle bones.

- What does the prefix "trans-" mean?
  Answer: Across or through - The prefix "trans-" indicates across or through. For example, "transdermal" refers to the administration of medication through the skin.

- What does the suffix "-ectomy" mean?
  Answer: Surgical removal - The suffix "-ectomy" denotes surgical removal. For example, "appendectomy" refers to the surgical removal of the appendix.

- What does the root word "myo" refer to?
  Answer: Muscle - The root word "myo" pertains to muscles. For example, "myopathy" refers to a disease of the muscle tissue.

- What does the prefix "hyper-" mean?
  Answer: Above normal or excessive - The prefix "hyper-" indicates above normal or excessive. For example, "hypertension" refers to abnormally high blood pressure.

- What does the suffix "-itis" mean?
  Answer: Inflammation - The suffix "-itis" denotes inflammation. For example, "tonsillitis" refers to the inflammation of the tonsils.

- What does the root word "neur" refer to?
  Answer: Nerve - The root word "neur" pertains to nerves. For example, "neurology" is the branch of medicine dealing with the nervous system and its disorders.

- What does the prefix "intra-" mean?
  Answer: Within - The prefix "intra-" indicates within. For example, "intravenous" refers to something administered within or into a vein.

- What does the suffix "-oma" mean?
  Answer: Tumor or mass - The suffix "-oma" denotes a tumor or mass. For example, "carcinoma" refers to a type of cancer that starts in the cells that make up the skin or the tissue lining organs.

- What does the root word "thorac" refer to?
  Answer: Chest - The root word "thorac" pertains to the chest. For example, "thoracotomy" refers to a surgical incision into the chest wall.

- What does the prefix "anti-" mean?
  Answer: Against - The prefix "anti-" indicates against. For example, "antibiotic" refers to a substance that works against bacteria.

- What does the suffix "-logy" mean?
  Answer: Study of - The suffix "-logy" denotes the study of. For example, "biology" is the study of living organisms.

- What does the root word "gastr" refer to?
  Answer: Stomach - The root word "gastr" pertains to the stomach. For example, "gastritis" refers to the inflammation of the stomach lining.

- What does the prefix "post-" mean?
  Answer: After - The prefix "post-" indicates after. For example, "postoperative" refers to the period after surgery.

- What does the suffix "-genic" mean?
  Answer: Producing or causing - The suffix "-genic" denotes producing or causing. For example, "carcinogenic" refers to something that produces or causes cancer.

- What does the prefix "sub-" mean?
  Answer: Under or below - The prefix "sub-" indicates under or below. For example, "subcutaneous" refers to something situated or applied under the skin.

- What does the suffix "-lysis" mean?
  Answer: Breakdown or destruction - The suffix "-lysis" denotes breakdown or destruction. For example, "hemolysis" refers to the destruction of red blood cells.

- What does the root word "cardi" refer to?
  Answer: Heart - The root word "cardi" pertains to the heart. For example, "cardiology" is the branch of medicine dealing with the heart and its diseases.

- What does the prefix "epi-" mean?
  Answer: Upon or above - The prefix "epi-" indicates upon or above. For example, "epidermis" refers to the outer layer of skin.

- What does the suffix "-pathy" mean?
  Answer: Disease or disorder - The suffix "-pathy" denotes disease or disorder. For example, "neuropathy" refers to a disease or dysfunction of one or more peripheral nerves.

- What does the root word "rhin" refer to?
  Answer: Nose - The root word "rhin" pertains to the nose. For example, "rhinitis" refers to the inflammation of the mucous membrane of the nose.

- What does the prefix "brady-" mean?
  Answer: Slow - The prefix "brady-" indicates slow. For example, "bradycardia" refers to a slower than normal heart rate.

- What does the suffix "-plasty" mean?
  Answer: Surgical repair - The suffix "-plasty" denotes surgical repair. For example, "rhinoplasty" refers to the surgical repair or reshaping of the nose.

- What does the root word "cephal" refer to?
  Answer: Head - The root word "cephal" pertains to the head. For example, "cephalalgia" refers to a headache.

- What does the prefix "tachy-" mean?
  Answer: Fast - The prefix "tachy-" indicates fast. For example, "tachycardia" refers to a faster than normal heart rate.

- What does the suffix "-rrhea" mean?
  Answer: Flow or discharge - The suffix "-rrhea" denotes flow or discharge. For example, "diarrhea" refers to the condition of having frequent and watery bowel movements.

- What does the root word "arthr" refer to?
  Answer: Joint - The root word "arthr" pertains to joints. For example, "arthritis" refers to the inflammation of one or more joints.

- What does the prefix "hypo-" mean?
  Answer: Below normal or deficient - The prefix "hypo-" indicates below normal or deficient. For example, "hypoglycemia" refers to abnormally low levels of glucose in the blood.

- What does the suffix "-scopy" mean?
  Answer: Visual examination - The suffix "-scopy" denotes visual examination. For example, "endoscopy" refers to a procedure in which an instrument is introduced into the body to give a view of its internal parts.

- What does the root word "cyt" refer to?
  Answer: Cell - The root word "cyt" pertains to cells. For example, "cytology" is the study of cells.

- What does the prefix "retro-" mean?
  Answer: Backward or behind - The prefix "retro-" indicates backward or behind. For example, "retroperitoneal" refers to the anatomical space in the abdominal cavity behind the peritoneum.

- What does the suffix "-tomy" mean?
  Answer: Cutting or incision - The suffix "-tomy" denotes cutting or incision. For example, "tracheotomy" refers to an incision in the windpipe made to relieve an obstruction to breathing.

- What does the root word "glyc" refer to?
  Answer: Sugar - The root word "glyc" pertains to sugar. For example, "glycemia" refers to the presence of glucose in the blood.

- What does the prefix "inter-" mean?
  Answer: Between - The prefix "inter-" indicates between. For example, "intercostal" refers to something situated between the ribs.

- What does the suffix "-uria" mean?
  Answer: Urine condition - The suffix "-uria" denotes a urine condition. For example, "hematuria" refers to the presence of blood in the urine.

- What does the root word "lip" refer to?
  Answer: Fat - The root word "lip" pertains to fat. For example, "liposuction" is a surgical procedure to remove fat from specific areas of the body.

- What does the suffix "-emia" mean?
  Answer: Blood condition - The suffix "-emia" denotes a blood condition. For example, "anemia" refers to a condition in which there is a deficiency of red cells or hemoglobin in the blood.

- What does the root word "nephr" refer to?
  Answer: Kidney - The root word "nephr" pertains to the kidney. For example, "nephrology" is the branch of medicine that deals with the physiology and diseases of the kidneys.

- What does the prefix "trans-" mean?
  Answer: Across or through - The prefix "trans-" indicates across or through. For example, "transdermal" refers to the administration of medication through the skin.

- What does the suffix "-genic" mean?
  Answer: Producing or causing - The suffix "-genic" denotes producing or causing. For example, "carcinogenic" refers to a substance capable of causing cancer.

- What does the root word "derm" refer to?
  Answer: Skin - The root word "derm" pertains to the skin. For example, "dermatology" is the branch of medicine dealing with the skin and its diseases.

- What does the prefix "poly-" mean?
  Answer: Many or much - The prefix "poly-" indicates many or much. For example, "polyuria" refers to the production of abnormally large volumes of dilute urine.

- What does the suffix "-stasis" mean?
  Answer: Stopping or controlling - The suffix "-stasis" denotes stopping or controlling. For example, "hemostasis" refers to the stopping of a flow of blood.

- What does the root word "hepat" refer to?
  Answer: Liver - The root word "hepat" pertains to the liver. For example, "hepatitis" refers to the inflammation of the liver.

- What does the prefix "auto-" mean?
  Answer: Self - The prefix "auto-" indicates self. For example, "autoimmune" refers to a condition in which the body's immune system attacks its own tissues.

- What does the suffix "-phobia" mean?
  Answer: Fear - The suffix "-phobia" denotes fear. For example, "claustrophobia" refers to the fear of confined spaces.

- What does the root word "oste" refer to?
  Answer: Bone - The root word "oste" pertains to bone. For example, "osteoporosis" refers to a condition in which bones become weak and brittle.

- What does the prefix "contra-" mean?
  Answer: Against or opposite - The prefix "contra-" indicates against or opposite. For example, "contraceptive" refers to a method or device serving to prevent pregnancy.

- What does the suffix "-ectomy" mean?
  Answer: Surgical removal - The suffix "-ectomy" denotes surgical removal. For example, "appendectomy" refers to the surgical removal of the appendix.

- What does the root word "myo" refer to?
  Answer: Muscle - The root word "myo" pertains to muscle. For example, "myopathy" refers to a disease of the muscle tissue.

- What does the prefix "hyper-" mean?
  Answer: Above normal or excessive - The prefix "hyper-" indicates above normal or excessive. For example, "hypertension" refers to abnormally high blood pressure.

- What does the suffix "-logy" mean?
  Answer: Study of - The suffix "-logy" denotes the study of. For example, "biology" is the study of living organisms.

- What does the root word "thorac" refer to?
  Answer: Chest - The root word "thorac" pertains to the chest. For example, "thoracic" refers to the part of the body between the neck and the abdomen.

- What does the prefix "infra-" mean?
  Answer: Below or beneath - The prefix "infra-" indicates below or beneath. For example, "infrared" refers to electromagnetic radiation with wavelengths longer than those of visible light, and thus below the red end of the spectrum.

- What does the suffix "-oma" mean?
  Answer: Tumor or mass - The suffix "-oma" denotes a tumor or mass. For example, "carcinoma" refers to a type of cancer that starts in cells that make up the skin or the tissue lining organs.

- What does the root word "encephal" refer to?
  Answer: Brain - The root word "encephal" pertains to the brain. For example, "encephalitis" refers to the inflammation of the brain.

- What does the suffix "-itis" mean?
  Answer: Inflammation - The suffix "-itis" denotes inflammation. For example, "arthritis" refers to the inflammation of the joints.

- What does the root word "cardi" refer to?
  Answer: Heart - The root word "cardi" pertains to the heart. For example, "cardiology" is the branch of medicine that deals with diseases and abnormalities of the heart.

- What does the prefix "epi-" mean?
  Answer: Upon or above - The prefix "epi-" indicates upon or above. For example, "epidermis" refers to the outer layer of skin cells.

- What does the suffix "-lysis" mean?
  Answer: Breakdown or destruction - The suffix "-lysis" denotes breakdown or destruction. For example, "hemolysis" refers to the destruction of red blood cells.

- What does the root word "gastr" refer to?
  Answer: Stomach - The root word "gastr" pertains to the stomach. For example, "gastritis" refers to the inflammation of the stomach lining.

- What does the prefix "hypo-" mean?
  Answer: Below normal or deficient - The prefix "hypo-" indicates below normal or deficient. For example, "hypoglycemia" refers to abnormally low levels of glucose in the blood.

- What does the suffix "-pathy" mean?
  Answer: Disease or disorder - The suffix "-pathy" denotes disease or disorder. For example, "neuropathy" refers to a disease or dysfunction of one or more peripheral nerves.

- What does the root word "pulmon" refer to?
  Answer: Lung - The root word "pulmon" pertains to the lung. For example, "pulmonology" is the branch of medicine that deals with diseases involving the respiratory tract.

- What does the prefix "inter-" mean?
  Answer: Between or among - The prefix "inter-" indicates between or among. For example, "intercellular" refers to something occurring between cells.

- What does the suffix "-rrhea" mean?
  Answer: Flow or discharge - The suffix "-rrhea" denotes flow or discharge. For example, "diarrhea" refers to the condition of having frequent and watery bowel movements.

- What does the root word "cephal" refer to?
  Answer: Head - The root word "cephal" pertains to the head. For example, "cephalalgia" refers to a headache.

- What does the prefix "retro-" mean?
  Answer: Backward or behind - The prefix "retro-" indicates backward or behind. For example, "retrograde" refers to moving backward.

- What does the suffix "-plasty" mean?
  Answer: Surgical repair - The suffix "-plasty" denotes surgical repair. For example, "rhinoplasty" refers to the surgical repair or reshaping of the nose.

- What does the root word "arthr" refer to?
  Answer: Joint - The root word "arthr" pertains to joints. For example, "arthritis" refers to the inflammation of one or more joints.

- What does the prefix "peri-" mean?
  Answer: Around or surrounding - The prefix "peri-" indicates around or surrounding. For example, "pericardium" refers to the membrane enclosing the heart.

- What does the suffix "-emia" mean?
  Answer: Blood condition - The suffix "-emia" denotes a blood condition. For example, "anemia" refers to a condition in which there is a deficiency of red cells or hemoglobin in the blood.

- What does the root word "nephr" refer to?
  Answer: Kidney - The root word "nephr" pertains to the kidney. For example, "nephrology" is the branch of medicine that deals with the physiology and diseases of the kidneys.

- What does the prefix "trans-" mean?
  Answer: Across or through - The prefix "trans-" indicates across or through. For example, "transdermal" refers to the administration of medication through the skin.

- What does the suffix "-genic" mean?
  Answer: Producing or causing - The suffix "-genic" denotes producing or causing. For example, "carcinogenic" refers to a substance capable of causing cancer.

- What does the root word "derm" refer to?
  Answer: Skin - The root word "derm" pertains to the skin. For example, "dermatology" is the branch of medicine dealing with the skin and its diseases.

- What does the prefix "poly-" mean?
  Answer: Many or much - The prefix "poly-" indicates many or much. For example, "polyuria" refers to the production of abnormally large volumes of dilute urine.

- What does the root word "hepat" refer to?
  Answer: Liver - The root word "hepat" pertains to the liver. For example, "hepatitis" refers to the inflammation of the liver.

- What does the prefix "brady-" mean?
  Answer: Slow - The prefix "brady-" indicates slowness. For example, "bradycardia" refers to a slower than normal heart rate.

- What does the suffix "-ectomy" mean?
  Answer: Surgical removal - The suffix "-ectomy" denotes surgical removal. For example, "appendectomy" refers to the surgical removal of the appendix.

- What does the root word "oste" refer to?
  Answer: Bone - The root word "oste" pertains to bones. For example, "osteoporosis" refers to a condition in which bones become weak and brittle.

- What does the prefix "tachy-" mean?
  Answer: Fast - The prefix "tachy-" indicates fast. For example, "tachycardia" refers to a faster than normal heart rate.

- What does the suffix "-graphy" mean?
  Answer: Process of recording - The suffix "-graphy" denotes the process of recording. For example, "angiography" refers to the imaging of blood vessels.

- What does the root word "myo" refer to?
  Answer: Muscle - The root word "myo" pertains to muscles. For example, "myopathy" refers to a disease of the muscle tissue.

- What does the prefix "hyper-" mean?
  Answer: Above normal or excessive - The prefix "hyper-" indicates above normal or excessive. For example, "hyperglycemia" refers to abnormally high levels of glucose in the blood.

- What does the suffix "-scopy" mean?
  Answer: Visual examination - The suffix "-scopy" denotes visual examination. For example, "endoscopy" refers to the examination of the interior of a body organ or cavity using a specialized instrument.

- What does the root word "neur" refer to?
  Answer: Nerve - The root word "neur" pertains to nerves. For example, "neurology" is the branch of medicine dealing with disorders of the nervous system.

- What does the prefix "intra-" mean?
  Answer: Within or inside - The prefix "intra-" indicates within or inside. For example, "intravenous" refers to something administered within or into a vein.

- What does the suffix "-oma" mean?
  Answer: Tumor or mass - The suffix "-oma" denotes a tumor or mass. For example, "carcinoma" refers to a type of cancer that begins in the skin or in tissues that line or cover internal organs.

- What does the root word "thorac" refer to?
  Answer: Chest - The root word "thorac" pertains to the chest. For example, "thoracotomy" refers to a surgical incision into the chest wall.

- What does the prefix "sub-" mean?
  Answer: Under or below - The prefix "sub-" indicates under or below. For example, "subcutaneous" refers to something situated or applied under the skin.

- What does the suffix "-logy" mean?
  Answer: Study of - The suffix "-logy" denotes the study of a particular subject. For example, "biology" refers to the study of living organisms.

- What does the root word "phleb" refer to?
  Answer: Vein - The root word "phleb" pertains to veins. For example, "phlebitis" refers to the inflammation of a vein.

- What does the prefix "anti-" mean?
  Answer: Against or opposing - The prefix "anti-" indicates against or opposing. For example, "antibiotic" refers to a substance that works against bacteria.

- What does the suffix "-phobia" mean?
  Answer: Fear - The suffix "-phobia" denotes fear. For example, "claustrophobia" refers to the fear of confined spaces.

- What does the root word "encephal" refer to?
  Answer: Brain - The root word "encephal" pertains to the brain. For example, "encephalitis" refers to the inflammation of the brain.

- What does the prefix "auto-" mean?
  Answer: Self - The prefix "auto-" indicates self. For example, "autoimmune" refers to a condition in which the body's immune system attacks its own tissues.

- What does the suffix "-tomy" mean?
  Answer: Cutting or incision - The suffix "-tomy" denotes cutting or incision. For example, "tracheotomy" refers to a surgical procedure to create an opening in the trachea.

- What does the prefix "peri-" mean?
  Answer: Around - The prefix "peri-" indicates around. For example, "pericardium" refers to the membrane surrounding the heart.

- What does the suffix "-lysis" mean?
  Answer: Breakdown or destruction - The suffix "-lysis" denotes breakdown or destruction. For example, "hemolysis" refers to the destruction of red blood cells.

- What does the root word "derm" refer to?
  Answer: Skin - The root word "derm" pertains to the skin. For example, "dermatology" is the branch of medicine dealing with the skin and its diseases.

- What does the prefix "hypo-" mean?
  Answer: Below normal or deficient - The prefix "hypo-" indicates below normal or deficient. For example, "hypoglycemia" refers to abnormally low levels of glucose in the blood.

- What does the suffix "-stasis" mean?
  Answer: Stopping or controlling - The suffix "-stasis" denotes stopping or controlling. For example, "hemostasis" refers to the process of stopping bleeding.

- What does the root word "cardi" refer to?
  Answer: Heart - The root word "cardi" pertains to the heart. For example, "cardiology" is the branch of medicine dealing with disorders of the heart.

- What does the prefix "epi-" mean?
  Answer: Upon or above - The prefix "epi-" indicates upon or above. For example, "epidermis" refers to the outer layer of skin.

- What does the suffix "-itis" mean?
  Answer: Inflammation - The suffix "-itis" denotes inflammation. For example, "arthritis" refers to the inflammation of the joints.

- What does the root word "gastr" refer to?
  Answer: Stomach - The root word "gastr" pertains to the stomach. For example, "gastritis" refers to the inflammation of the stomach lining.

- What does the prefix "poly-" mean?
  Answer: Many or much - The prefix "poly-" indicates many or much. For example, "polyuria" refers to the production of abnormally large volumes of urine.

- What does the suffix "-pathy" mean?
  Answer: Disease or disorder - The suffix "-pathy" denotes disease or disorder. For example, "neuropathy" refers to a disease or dysfunction of one or more peripheral nerves.

- What does the root word "nephr" refer to?
  Answer: Kidney - The root word "nephr" pertains to the kidneys. For example, "nephrology" is the branch of medicine that deals with the physiology and diseases of the kidneys.

- What does the prefix "trans-" mean?
  Answer: Across or through - The prefix "trans-" indicates across or through. For example, "transdermal" refers to the administration of medication through the skin.

- What does the suffix "-emia" mean?
  Answer: Blood condition - The suffix "-emia" denotes a blood condition. For example, "anemia" refers to a condition in which there is a deficiency of red cells or of hemoglobin in the blood.

- What does the root word "arthr" refer to?
  Answer: Joint - The root word "arthr" pertains to joints. For example, "arthritis" refers to the inflammation of the joints.

- What does the prefix "inter-" mean?
  Answer: Between - The prefix "inter-" indicates between. For example, "intercostal" refers to something situated between the ribs.

- What does the suffix "-plasty" mean?
  Answer: Surgical repair - The suffix "-plasty" denotes surgical repair. For example, "rhinoplasty" refers to the surgical repair or reshaping of the nose.

- What does the root word "cyt" refer to?
  Answer: Cell - The root word "cyt" pertains to cells. For example, "cytology" is the branch of biology concerned with the structure and function of plant and animal cells.

- What does the prefix "retro-" mean?
  Answer: Backward or behind - The prefix "retro-" indicates backward or behind. For example, "retroperitoneal" refers to the anatomical space in the abdominal cavity behind the peritoneum.

- What does the suffix "-rrhea" mean?
  Answer: Flow or discharge - The suffix "-rrhea" denotes flow or discharge. For example, "diarrhea" refers to the condition of having frequent and liquid bowel movements.

- What does the root word "hemat" refer to?
  Answer: Blood - The root word "hemat" pertains to blood. For example, "hematology" is the branch of medicine concerned with the study of blood, blood-forming organs, and blood diseases.

- What does the suffix "-ectomy" mean?
  Answer: Surgical removal - The suffix "-ectomy" denotes surgical removal. For example, "appendectomy" refers to the surgical removal of the appendix.

- What does the root word "myo" refer to?
  Answer: Muscle - The root word "myo" pertains to muscles. For example, "myopathy" refers to a disease of muscle tissue.

- What does the prefix "tachy-" mean?
  Answer: Fast or rapid - The prefix "tachy-" indicates fast or rapid. For example, "tachycardia" refers to an abnormally rapid heart rate.

- What does the suffix "-genesis" mean?
  Answer: Formation or origin - The suffix "-genesis" denotes formation or origin. For example, "osteogenesis" refers to the formation of bone.

- What does the root word "neur" refer to?
  Answer: Nerve - The root word "neur" pertains to nerves. For example, "neurology" is the branch of medicine dealing with disorders of the nervous system.

- What does the prefix "brady-" mean?
  Answer: Slow - The prefix "brady-" indicates slow. For example, "bradycardia" refers to an abnormally slow heart rate.

- What does the suffix "-phobia" mean?
  Answer: Fear - The suffix "-phobia" denotes fear. For example, "claustrophobia" refers to the fear of confined spaces.

- What does the root word "hepat" refer to?
  Answer: Liver - The root word "hepat" pertains to the liver. For example, "hepatitis" refers to the inflammation of the liver.

- What does the prefix "anti-" mean?
  Answer: Against - The prefix "anti-" indicates against. For example, "antibiotic" refers to a substance that works against bacteria.

- What does the suffix "-logy" mean?
  Answer: Study of - The suffix "-logy" denotes the study of. For example, "biology" refers to the study of living organisms.

- What does the root word "oste" refer to?
  Answer: Bone - The root word "oste" pertains to bones. For example, "osteoporosis" refers to a condition in which bones become weak and brittle.

- What does the prefix "auto-" mean?
  Answer: Self - The prefix "auto-" indicates self. For example, "autoimmune" refers to a condition in which the body's immune system attacks its own tissues.

- What does the suffix "-oma" mean?
  Answer: Tumor or mass - The suffix "-oma" denotes a tumor or mass. For example, "carcinoma" refers to a type of cancer that begins in the skin or in tissues that line or cover internal organs.

- What does the root word "thorac" refer to?
  Answer: Chest - The root word "thorac" pertains to the chest. For example, "thoracic" refers to the part of the body between the neck and the abdomen.

- What does the prefix "hyper-" mean?
  Answer: Above normal or excessive - The prefix "hyper-" indicates above normal or excessive. For example, "hypertension" refers to abnormally high blood pressure.

- What does the suffix "-scope" mean?
  Answer: Instrument for viewing - The suffix "-scope" denotes an instrument for viewing. For example, "microscope" refers to an instrument used to see objects that are too small to be seen by the naked eye.

- What does the root word "angi" refer to?
  Answer: Vessel - The root word "angi" pertains to vessels. For example, "angioplasty" refers to the surgical repair or unblocking of a blood vessel.

- What does the prefix "peri-" mean?
  Answer: Around - The prefix "peri-" indicates around. For example, "pericardium" refers to the membrane surrounding the heart.

- What does the suffix "-lysis" mean?
  Answer: Breakdown or destruction - The suffix "-lysis" denotes breakdown or destruction. For example, "hemolysis" refers to the destruction of red blood cells.

- What does the root word "derm" refer to?
  Answer: Skin - The root word "derm" pertains to the skin. For example, "dermatology" is the branch of medicine dealing with the skin and its diseases.

- What does the prefix "hypo-" mean?
  Answer: Below normal or deficient - The prefix "hypo-" indicates below normal or deficient. For example, "hypoglycemia" refers to abnormally low levels of glucose in the blood.

- What does the root word "cardi" refer to?
  Answer: Heart - The root word "cardi" pertains to the heart. For example, "cardiology" is the branch of medicine dealing with disorders of the heart.

- What does the prefix "poly-" mean?
  Answer: Many - The prefix "poly-" indicates many. For example, "polyuria" refers to the production of abnormally large volumes of dilute urine.

- What does the suffix "-itis" mean?
  Answer: Inflammation - The suffix "-itis" denotes inflammation. For example, "arthritis" refers to inflammation of the joints.

- What does the root word "gastr" refer to?
  Answer: Stomach - The root word "gastr" pertains to the stomach. For example, "gastritis" refers to inflammation of the stomach lining.

- What does the prefix "sub-" mean?
  Answer: Under or below - The prefix "sub-" indicates under or below. For example, "subcutaneous" refers to something situated or applied under the skin.

- What does the suffix "-pathy" mean?
  Answer: Disease or disorder - The suffix "-pathy" denotes disease or disorder. For example, "neuropathy" refers to a disease or dysfunction of one or more peripheral nerves.

- What does the root word "ren" refer to?
  Answer: Kidney - The root word "ren" pertains to the kidneys. For example, "renal" refers to anything related to the kidneys.

- What does the prefix "epi-" mean?
  Answer: Upon or above - The prefix "epi-" indicates upon or above. For example, "epidermis" refers to the outer layer of skin cells.

- What does the suffix "-plasty" mean?
  Answer: Surgical repair - The suffix "-plasty" denotes surgical repair. For example, "rhinoplasty" refers to the surgical repair or reshaping of the nose.

- What does the root word "cephal" refer to?
  Answer: Head - The root word "cephal" pertains to the head. For example, "cephalalgia" refers to a headache.

- What does the prefix "endo-" mean?
  Answer: Within or inside - The prefix "endo-" indicates within or inside. For example, "endoscopy" refers to a procedure that allows doctors to view the inside of the body.

- What does the suffix "-emia" mean?
  Answer: Blood condition - The suffix "-emia" denotes a blood condition. For example, "anemia" refers to a condition in which there is a deficiency of red cells or of hemoglobin in the blood.

- What does the root word "arthr" refer to?
  Answer: Joint - The root word "arthr" pertains to joints. For example, "arthritis" refers to inflammation of the joints.

- What does the prefix "inter-" mean?
  Answer: Between - The prefix "inter-" indicates between. For example, "intercostal" refers to something situated between the ribs.

- What does the suffix "-graphy" mean?
  Answer: Process of recording - The suffix "-graphy" denotes the process of recording. For example, "angiography" refers to the imaging of blood vessels.

- What does the root word "cyt" refer to?
  Answer: Cell - The root word "cyt" pertains to cells. For example, "cytology" is the study of cells.

- What does the prefix "trans-" mean?
  Answer: Across or through - The prefix "trans-" indicates across or through. For example, "transdermal" refers to something administered across the skin.

- What does the suffix "-tomy" mean?
  Answer: Cutting or incision - The suffix "-tomy" denotes cutting or incision. For example, "tracheotomy" refers to an incision in the windpipe made to relieve an obstruction to breathing.

- What does the root word "hem" refer to?
  Answer: Blood - The root word "hem" pertains to blood. For example, "hemorrhage" refers to an escape of blood from a ruptured blood vessel.

- What does the prefix "retro-" mean?
  Answer: Backward or behind - The prefix "retro-" indicates backward or behind. For example, "retroperitoneal" refers to something situated behind the peritoneum.

- What does the suffix "-megaly" mean?
  Answer: Enlargement - The suffix "-megaly" denotes enlargement. For example, "cardiomegaly" refers to the enlargement of the heart.

- What does the prefix "hypo-" mean?
  Answer: Under or below normal - The prefix "hypo-" indicates under or below normal. For example, "hypoglycemia" refers to abnormally low levels of glucose in the blood.

- What does the suffix "-lysis" mean?
  Answer: Breakdown or destruction - The suffix "-lysis" denotes breakdown or destruction. For example, "hemolysis" refers to the destruction of red blood cells.

- What does the root word "derm" refer to?
  Answer: Skin - The root word "derm" pertains to the skin. For example, "dermatology" is the branch of medicine dealing with the skin and its diseases.

- What does the prefix "peri-" mean?
  Answer: Around or surrounding - The prefix "peri-" indicates around or surrounding. For example, "pericardium" refers to the membrane enclosing the heart.

- What does the suffix "-oma" mean?
  Answer: Tumor or mass - The suffix "-oma" denotes a tumor or mass. For example, "carcinoma" refers to a type of cancer that begins in the skin or in tissues that line or cover internal organs.

- What does the root word "myo" refer to?
  Answer: Muscle - The root word "myo" pertains to muscles. For example, "myopathy" refers to a disease of the muscle tissue.

- What does the prefix "tachy-" mean?
  Answer: Fast or rapid - The prefix "tachy-" indicates fast or rapid. For example, "tachycardia" refers to an abnormally rapid heart rate.

- What does the suffix "-stasis" mean?
  Answer: Stopping or controlling - The suffix "-stasis" denotes stopping or controlling. For example, "hemostasis" refers to the process of stopping bleeding.

- What does the root word "oste" refer to?
  Answer: Bone - The root word "oste" pertains to bones. For example, "osteoporosis" refers to a condition in which bones become weak and brittle.

- What does the prefix "brady-" mean?
  Answer: Slow - The prefix "brady-" indicates slow. For example, "bradycardia" refers to an abnormally slow heart rate.

- What does the suffix "-ectomy" mean?
  Answer: Surgical removal - The suffix "-ectomy" denotes surgical removal. For example, "appendectomy" refers to the surgical removal of the appendix.

- What does the root word "neur" refer to?
  Answer: Nerve - The root word "neur" pertains to nerves. For example, "neurology" is the branch of medicine dealing with disorders of the nervous system.

- What does the prefix "hyper-" mean?
  Answer: Over or above normal - The prefix "hyper-" indicates over or above normal. For example, "hypertension" refers to abnormally high blood pressure.

- What does the suffix "-scopy" mean?
  Answer: Visual examination - The suffix "-scopy" denotes visual examination. For example, "endoscopy" refers to a procedure that allows doctors to view the inside of the body.

- What does the root word "hepat" refer to?
  Answer: Liver - The root word "hepat" pertains to the liver. For example, "hepatitis" refers to inflammation of the liver.

- What does the prefix "intra-" mean?
  Answer: Within or inside - The prefix "intra-" indicates within or inside. For example, "intravenous" refers to something administered within or into a vein.

- What does the suffix "-algia" mean?
  Answer: Pain - The suffix "-algia" denotes pain. For example, "neuralgia" refers to intense, typically intermittent pain along the course of a nerve.

- What does the root word "pulmon" refer to?
  Answer: Lung - The root word "pulmon" pertains to the lungs. For example, "pulmonology" is the branch of medicine dealing with diseases involving the respiratory tract.

- What does the prefix "anti-" mean?
  Answer: Against - The prefix "anti-" indicates against. For example, "antibiotic" refers to a substance that works against bacteria.

- What does the suffix "-genic" mean?
  Answer: Producing or causing - The suffix "-genic" denotes producing or causing. For example, "carcinogenic" refers to something that produces or causes cancer.

- What does the root word "thorac" refer to?
  Answer: Chest - The root word "thorac" pertains to the chest. For example, "thoracic" refers to anything related to the chest area.

- What does the prefix "auto-" mean?
  Answer: Self - The prefix "auto-" indicates self. For example, "autoimmune" refers to a condition in which the body's immune system attacks its own tissues.

- What does the prefix "sub-" mean?
  Answer: Under or below - The prefix "sub-" indicates under or below. For example, "subcutaneous" refers to something situated or applied under the skin.

- What does the suffix "-phobia" mean?
  Answer: Fear - The suffix "-phobia" denotes fear. For example, "arachnophobia" refers to an intense fear of spiders.

- What does the root word "cardi" refer to?
  Answer: Heart - The root word "cardi" pertains to the heart. For example, "cardiology" is the branch of medicine dealing with disorders of the heart.

- What does the prefix "epi-" mean?
  Answer: Upon or above - The prefix "epi-" indicates upon or above. For example, "epidermis" refers to the outer layer of skin.

- What does the suffix "-itis" mean?
  Answer: Inflammation - The suffix "-itis" denotes inflammation. For example, "arthritis" refers to inflammation of the joints.

- What does the root word "gastr" refer to?
  Answer: Stomach - The root word "gastr" pertains to the stomach. For example, "gastritis" refers to inflammation of the stomach lining.

- What does the prefix "poly-" mean?
  Answer: Many - The prefix "poly-" indicates many. For example, "polyuria" refers to the production of abnormally large volumes of dilute urine.

- What does the suffix "-cyte" mean?
  Answer: Cell - The suffix "-cyte" denotes a cell. For example, "erythrocyte" refers to a red blood cell.

- What does the root word "encephal" refer to?
  Answer: Brain - The root word "encephal" pertains to the brain. For example, "encephalitis" refers to inflammation of the brain.

- What does the prefix "retro-" mean?
  Answer: Backward or behind - The prefix "retro-" indicates backward or behind. For example, "retrograde" refers to moving backward.

- What does the suffix "-plasty" mean?
  Answer: Surgical repair - The suffix "-plasty" denotes surgical repair. For example, "rhinoplasty" refers to the surgical repair or reshaping of the nose.

- What does the root word "cyt" refer to?
  Answer: Cell - The root word "cyt" pertains to cells. For example, "cytology" is the study of cells.

- What does the prefix "trans-" mean?
  Answer: Across or through - The prefix "trans-" indicates across or through. For example, "transdermal" refers to something administered across the skin.

- What does the suffix "-emia" mean?
  Answer: Blood condition - The suffix "-emia" denotes a blood condition. For example, "anemia" refers to a condition in which there is a deficiency of red cells or hemoglobin in the blood.

- What does the root word "nephr" refer to?
  Answer: Kidney - The root word "nephr" pertains to the kidneys. For example, "nephrology" is the branch of medicine that deals with the physiology and diseases of the kidneys.

- What does the prefix "inter-" mean?
  Answer: Between - The prefix "inter-" indicates between. For example, "intercostal" refers to something situated between the ribs.

- What does the suffix "-graphy" mean?
  Answer: Process of recording - The suffix "-graphy" denotes the process of recording. For example, "angiography" refers to the imaging of blood vessels.

- What does the root word "phleb" refer to?
  Answer: Vein - The root word "phleb" pertains to veins. For example, "phlebitis" refers to inflammation of a vein.

- What does the prefix "pseudo-" mean?
  Answer: False - The prefix "pseudo-" indicates false. For example, "pseudocyst" refers to a false cyst.

- What does the suffix "-logy" mean?
  Answer: Study of - The suffix "-logy" denotes the study of. For example, "biology" refers to the study of living organisms.

- What does the root word "splen" refer to?
  Answer: Spleen - The root word "splen" pertains to the spleen. For example, "splenomegaly" refers to the enlargement of the spleen.

- What does the prefix "peri-" mean?
  Answer: Around or surrounding - The prefix "peri-" indicates around or surrounding. For example, "pericardium" refers to the membrane enclosing the heart.

- What does the suffix "-tomy" mean?
  Answer: Cutting or incision - The suffix "-tomy" denotes cutting or incision. For example, "tracheotomy" refers to an incision in the windpipe

- What does the prefix "brady-" mean?
  Answer: Slow - The prefix "brady-" indicates slowness. For example, "bradycardia" refers to a slower than normal heart rate.

- What does the suffix "-ectomy" mean?
  Answer: Surgical removal - The suffix "-ectomy" denotes the surgical removal of a part of the body. For example, "appendectomy" is the surgical removal of the appendix.

- What does the root word "hepat" refer to?
  Answer: Liver - The root word "hepat" pertains to the liver. For example, "hepatitis" refers to inflammation of the liver.

- What does the prefix "tachy-" mean?
  Answer: Fast - The prefix "tachy-" indicates fast. For example, "tachycardia" refers to a faster than normal heart rate.

- What does the suffix "-algia" mean?
  Answer: Pain - The suffix "-algia" denotes pain. For example, "neuralgia" refers to nerve pain.

- What does the root word "derm" refer to?
  Answer: Skin - The root word "derm" pertains to the skin. For example, "dermatology" is the study of skin and its diseases.

- What does the prefix "hyper-" mean?
  Answer: Excessive or above normal - The prefix "hyper-" indicates excessive or above normal. For example, "hypertension" refers to abnormally high blood pressure.

- What does the suffix "-scopy" mean?
  Answer: Visual examination - The suffix "-scopy" denotes visual examination. For example, "endoscopy" refers to the visual examination of the interior of a body organ or cavity.

- What does the root word "oste" refer to?
  Answer: Bone - The root word "oste" pertains to bones. For example, "osteoporosis" refers to a condition characterized by weak and brittle bones.

- What does the prefix "hypo-" mean?
  Answer: Below normal or deficient - The prefix "hypo-" indicates below normal or deficient. For example, "hypoglycemia" refers to low blood sugar levels.

- What does the suffix "-megaly" mean?
  Answer: Enlargement - The suffix "-megaly" denotes enlargement. For example, "cardiomegaly" refers to the enlargement of the heart.

- What does the root word "neur" refer to?
  Answer: Nerve - The root word "neur" pertains to nerves. For example, "neurology" is the study of the nervous system and its disorders.

- What does the prefix "peri-" mean?
  Answer: Around or surrounding - The prefix "peri-" indicates around or surrounding. For example, "pericardium" refers to the membrane surrounding the heart.

- What does the suffix "-stasis" mean?
  Answer: Stopping or controlling - The suffix "-stasis" denotes stopping or controlling. For example, "hemostasis" refers to the stopping of bleeding.

- What does the root word "gastr" refer to?
  Answer: Stomach - The root word "gastr" pertains to the stomach. For example, "gastritis" refers to inflammation of the stomach lining.

- What does the prefix "endo-" mean?
  Answer: Within or inside - The prefix "endo-" indicates within or inside. For example, "endocrine" refers to glands that secrete hormones directly into the bloodstream.

- What does the suffix "-lysis" mean?
  Answer: Breakdown or destruction - The suffix "-lysis" denotes breakdown or destruction. For example, "hemolysis" refers to the destruction of red blood cells.

- What does the root word "arthr" refer to?
  Answer: Joint - The root word "arthr" pertains to joints. For example, "arthritis" refers to inflammation of the joints.

- What does the prefix "exo-" mean?
  Answer: Outside or external - The prefix "exo-" indicates outside or external. For example, "exocrine" refers to glands that secrete substances through ducts to an external or internal surface.

- What does the suffix "-oma" mean?
  Answer: Tumor or mass - The suffix "-oma" denotes a tumor or mass. For example, "carcinoma" refers to a type of cancerous tumor.

- What does the root word "cardi" refer to?
  Answer: Heart - The root word "cardi" pertains to the heart. For example, "cardiology" is the study of the heart and its diseases.

- What does the prefix "intra-" mean?
  Answer: Within or inside - The prefix "intra-" indicates within or inside. For example, "intravenous" refers to something administered within a vein.

- What does the suffix "-pathy" mean?
  Answer: Disease or disorder - The suffix "-pathy" denotes disease or disorder. For example

- What does the suffix "-pathy" mean?
  Answer: Disease or disorder - The suffix "-pathy" denotes disease or disorder. For example, "neuropathy" refers to a disease or dysfunction of one or more peripheral nerves.

- What does the root word "pulmon" refer to?
  Answer: Lung - The root word "pulmon" pertains to the lungs. For example, "pulmonology" is the study of lung diseases and conditions.

- What does the prefix "sub-" mean?
  Answer: Under or below - The prefix "sub-" indicates under or below. For example, "subcutaneous" refers to something situated or applied under the skin.

- What does the suffix "-plasty" mean?
  Answer: Surgical repair - The suffix "-plasty" denotes surgical repair. For example, "rhinoplasty" refers to the surgical repair or reshaping of the nose.

- What does the root word "nephr" refer to?
  Answer: Kidney - The root word "nephr" pertains to the kidneys. For example, "nephrology" is the study of kidney function and diseases.

- What does the prefix "anti-" mean?
  Answer: Against or opposing - The prefix "anti-" indicates against or opposing. For example, "antibiotic" refers to a substance that works against bacteria.

- What does the suffix "-emia" mean?
  Answer: Blood condition - The suffix "-emia" denotes a blood condition. For example, "anemia" refers to a condition characterized by a deficiency of red blood cells or hemoglobin.

- What does the root word "encephal" refer to?
  Answer: Brain - The root word "encephal" pertains to the brain. For example, "encephalitis" refers to inflammation of the brain.

- What does the prefix "auto-" mean?
  Answer: Self - The prefix "auto-" indicates self. For example, "autoimmune" refers to a condition in which the body's immune system attacks its own tissues.

- What does the suffix "-graphy" mean?
  Answer: Process of recording - The suffix "-graphy" denotes the process of recording. For example, "angiography" refers to the imaging of blood vessels.

- What does the root word "cyt" refer to?
  Answer: Cell - The root word "cyt" pertains to cells. For example, "cytology" is the study of cells.

- What does the prefix "trans-" mean?
  Answer: Across or through - The prefix "trans-" indicates across or through. For example, "transdermal" refers to something administered across the skin.

- What does the suffix "-itis" mean?
  Answer: Inflammation - The suffix "-itis" denotes inflammation. For example, "tonsillitis" refers to inflammation of the tonsils.

- What does the root word "hemat" refer to?
  Answer: Blood - The root word "hemat" pertains to blood. For example, "hematology" is the study of blood and its disorders.

- What does the prefix "inter-" mean?
  Answer: Between - The prefix "inter-" indicates between. For example, "intercostal" refers to something situated between the ribs.

- What does the suffix "-rrhea" mean?
  Answer: Flow or discharge - The suffix "-rrhea" denotes flow or discharge. For example, "diarrhea" refers to the frequent flow of loose or liquid stools.

- What does the root word "myo" refer to?
  Answer: Muscle - The root word "myo" pertains to muscles. For example, "myopathy" refers to a disease of the muscle tissue.

- What does the prefix "poly-" mean?
  Answer: Many or much - The prefix "poly-" indicates many or much. For example, "polyuria" refers to the production of abnormally large volumes of urine.

- What does the suffix "-genesis" mean?
  Answer: Formation or production - The suffix "-genesis" denotes formation or production. For example, "osteogenesis" refers to the formation of bone.

- What does the root word "thorac" refer to?
  Answer: Chest - The root word "thorac" pertains to the chest. For example, "thoracotomy" refers to a surgical incision into the chest wall.

- What does the prefix "pre-" mean?
  Answer: Before - The prefix "pre-" indicates before. For example, "prenatal" refers to the period before birth.

- What does the suffix "-phobia" mean?
  Answer: Fear - The suffix "-phobia" denotes fear. For example, "claustrophobia" refers to the fear of confined spaces.

- What does the root word "glyc" refer to?
  Answer: Sugar - The root word "glyc" pertains to sugar. For example, "hyperglycemia" refers to high blood sugar levels.

- What does the prefix "peri-" mean?
  Answer: Around or surrounding - The prefix "peri-" indicates around or surrounding. For example, "pericardium" refers to the membrane surrounding the heart.

- What does the suffix "-lysis" mean?
  Answer: Breakdown or destruction - The suffix "-lysis" denotes breakdown or destruction. For example, "hemolysis" refers to the destruction of red blood cells.

- What does the root word "derm" refer to?
  Answer: Skin - The root word "derm" pertains to the skin. For example, "dermatology" is the study of skin and its diseases.

- What does the prefix "hypo-" mean?
  Answer: Under or below normal - The prefix "hypo-" indicates under or below normal. For example, "hypoglycemia" refers to low blood sugar levels.

- What does the suffix "-oma" mean?
  Answer: Tumor or mass - The suffix "-oma" denotes a tumor or mass. For example, "carcinoma" refers to a type of cancerous tumor.

- What does the root word "cardi" refer to?
  Answer: Heart - The root word "cardi" pertains to the heart. For example, "cardiology" is the study of heart diseases and conditions.

- What does the prefix "epi-" mean?
  Answer: Upon or above - The prefix "epi-" indicates upon or above. For example, "epidermis" refers to the outer layer of skin.

- What does the suffix "-stomy" mean?
  Answer: Creation of an opening - The suffix "-stomy" denotes the creation of an opening. For example, "colostomy" refers to the surgical creation of an opening in the colon.

- What does the root word "oste" refer to?
  Answer: Bone - The root word "oste" pertains to bones. For example, "osteoporosis" refers to a condition characterized by weakened bones.

- What does the prefix "hyper-" mean?
  Answer: Over or above normal - The prefix "hyper-" indicates over or above normal. For example, "hypertension" refers to high blood pressure.

- What does the suffix "-ectomy" mean?
  Answer: Surgical removal - The suffix "-ectomy" denotes surgical removal. For example, "appendectomy" refers to the surgical removal of the appendix.

- What does the root word "gastr" refer to?
  Answer: Stomach - The root word "gastr" pertains to the stomach. For example, "gastritis" refers to inflammation of the stomach lining.

- What does the prefix "retro-" mean?
  Answer: Backward or behind - The prefix "retro-" indicates backward or behind. For example, "retrograde" refers to moving backward.

- What does the suffix "-logy" mean?
  Answer: Study of - The suffix "-logy" denotes the study of a subject. For example, "biology" refers to the study of living organisms.

- What does the root word "hepat" refer to?
  Answer: Liver - The root word "hepat" pertains to the liver. For example, "hepatitis" refers to inflammation of the liver.

- What does the prefix "pseudo-" mean?
  Answer: False or deceptive - The prefix "pseudo-" indicates false or deceptive. For example, "pseudoscience" refers to a collection of beliefs mistakenly regarded as being based on scientific method.

- What does the suffix "-therapy" mean?
  Answer: Treatment - The suffix "-therapy" denotes treatment. For example, "chemotherapy" refers to the treatment of disease, especially cancer, using chemical substances.

- What does the root word "arthr" refer to?
  Answer: Joint - The root word "arthr" pertains to joints. For example, "arthritis" refers to inflammation of the joints.

- What does the prefix "tachy-" mean?
  Answer: Fast or rapid - The prefix "tachy-" indicates fast or rapid. For example, "tachycardia" refers to an abnormally rapid heart rate.

- What does the suffix "-scope" mean?
  Answer: Instrument for viewing - The suffix "-scope" denotes an instrument for viewing. For example, "microscope" refers to an instrument used to see objects that are too small for the naked eye.

- What does the root word "neur" refer to?
  Answer: Nerve - The root word "neur" pertains to nerves. For example, "neurology" is the study of the nervous system and its disorders.

- What does the prefix "brady-" mean?
  Answer: Slow - The prefix "brady-" indicates slow. For example, "bradycardia" refers to an abnormally slow heart rate.

- What does the root word "pulmon" refer to?
  Answer: Lung - The root word "pulmon" pertains to the lungs. For example, "pulmonology" is the study of lung diseases and conditions.

- What does the prefix "poly-" mean?
  Answer: Many or multiple - The prefix "poly-" indicates many or multiple. For example, "polyuria" refers to the production of abnormally large volumes of urine.

- What does the suffix "-phobia" mean?
  Answer: Fear - The suffix "-phobia" denotes fear. For example, "arachnophobia" refers to the fear of spiders.

- What does the root word "cephal" refer to?
  Answer: Head - The root word "cephal" pertains to the head. For example, "cephalalgia" refers to a headache.

- What does the prefix "auto-" mean?
  Answer: Self - The prefix "auto-" indicates self. For example, "autoimmune" refers to a condition where the body's immune system attacks its own tissues.

- What does the suffix "-genesis" mean?
  Answer: Formation or origin - The suffix "-genesis" denotes formation or origin. For example, "osteogenesis" refers to the formation of bone.

- What does the root word "myo" refer to?
  Answer: Muscle - The root word "myo" pertains to muscles. For example, "myopathy" refers to a disease of the muscle.

- What does the prefix "contra-" mean?
  Answer: Against or opposite - The prefix "contra-" indicates against or opposite. For example, "contraceptive" refers to a method or device serving to prevent pregnancy.

- What does the suffix "-itis" mean?
  Answer: Inflammation - The suffix "-itis" denotes inflammation. For example, "tonsillitis" refers to inflammation of the tonsils.

- What does the root word "nephr" refer to?
  Answer: Kidney - The root word "nephr" pertains to the kidneys. For example, "nephrology" is the study of kidney function and diseases.

- What does the prefix "inter-" mean?
  Answer: Between or among - The prefix "inter-" indicates between or among. For example, "intercellular" refers to something occurring between cells.

- What does the suffix "-cyte" mean?
  Answer: Cell - The suffix "-cyte" denotes a cell. For example, "erythrocyte" refers to a red blood cell.

- What does the root word "encephal" refer to?
  Answer: Brain - The root word "encephal" pertains to the brain. For example, "encephalitis" refers to inflammation of the brain.

- What does the prefix "trans-" mean?
  Answer: Across or through - The prefix "trans-" indicates across or through. For example, "transdermal" refers to something administered across the skin.

- What does the suffix "-oma" mean?
  Answer: Tumor or mass - The suffix "-oma" denotes a tumor or mass. For example, "melanoma" refers to a type of skin cancer.

- What does the root word "hemo" refer to?
  Answer: Blood - The root word "hemo" pertains to blood. For example, "hemoglobin" is the protein in red blood cells that carries oxygen.

- What does the prefix "peri-" mean?
  Answer: Around or surrounding - The prefix "peri-" indicates around or surrounding. For example, "perinatal" refers to the time period around birth.

- What does the suffix "-plasty" mean?
  Answer: Surgical repair - The suffix "-plasty" denotes surgical repair. For example, "rhinoplasty" refers to the surgical repair or reshaping of the nose.

- What does the root word "chondr" refer to?
  Answer: Cartilage - The root word "chondr" pertains to cartilage. For example, "chondritis" refers to inflammation of the cartilage.

- What does the prefix "sub-" mean?
  Answer: Under or below - The prefix "sub-" indicates under or below. For example, "subcutaneous" refers to something situated or applied under the skin.

- What does the suffix "-rrhea" mean?
  Answer: Flow or discharge - The suffix "-rrhea" denotes flow or discharge. For example, "diarrhea" refers to the condition of having frequent and fluid bowel movements.

- What does the root word "cyt" refer to?
  Answer: Cell - The root word "cyt" pertains to cells. For example, "cytology" is the study of cells.

- What does the suffix "-ectomy" mean?
  Answer: Surgical removal - The suffix "-ectomy" denotes surgical removal. For example, "appendectomy" refers to the surgical removal of the appendix.

- What does the root word "derm" refer to?
  Answer: Skin - The root word "derm" pertains to the skin. For example, "dermatology" is the study of skin and its diseases.

- What does the prefix "hyper-" mean?
  Answer: Excessive or above normal - The prefix "hyper-" indicates excessive or above normal. For example, "hypertension" refers to abnormally high blood pressure.

- What does the suffix "-logy" mean?
  Answer: Study of - The suffix "-logy" denotes the study of a particular subject. For example, "biology" is the study of living organisms.

- What does the root word "gastr" refer to?
  Answer: Stomach - The root word "gastr" pertains to the stomach. For example, "gastritis" refers to inflammation of the stomach lining.

- What does the prefix "hypo-" mean?
  Answer: Below normal or deficient - The prefix "hypo-" indicates below normal or deficient. For example, "hypoglycemia" refers to abnormally low blood sugar levels.

- What does the suffix "-pathy" mean?
  Answer: Disease or disorder - The suffix "-pathy" denotes disease or disorder. For example, "neuropathy" refers to a disease or dysfunction of the nerves.

- What does the root word "hepat" refer to?
  Answer: Liver - The root word "hepat" pertains to the liver. For example, "hepatitis" refers to inflammation of the liver.

- What does the prefix "epi-" mean?
  Answer: Upon or above - The prefix "epi-" indicates upon or above. For example, "epidermis" refers to the outer layer of skin.

- What does the suffix "-lysis" mean?
  Answer: Breakdown or destruction - The suffix "-lysis" denotes breakdown or destruction. For example, "hemolysis" refers to the destruction of red blood cells.

- What does the root word "oste" refer to?
  Answer: Bone - The root word "oste" pertains to bones. For example, "osteoporosis" refers to a condition characterized by weakened bones.

- What does the prefix "brady-" mean?
  Answer: Slow - The prefix "brady-" indicates slow. For example, "bradycardia" refers to a slower than normal heart rate.

- What does the suffix "-stomy" mean?
  Answer: Creating an opening - The suffix "-stomy" denotes creating an opening. For example, "colostomy" refers to the surgical creation of an opening in the colon.

- What does the root word "neur" refer to?
  Answer: Nerve - The root word "neur" pertains to nerves. For example, "neurology" is the study of the nervous system and its disorders.

- What does the prefix "tachy-" mean?
  Answer: Fast - The prefix "tachy-" indicates fast. For example, "tachycardia" refers to a faster than normal heart rate.

- What does the suffix "-graphy" mean?
  Answer: Process of recording - The suffix "-graphy" denotes the process of recording. For example, "angiography" refers to the imaging of blood vessels.

- What does the root word "phleb" refer to?
  Answer: Vein - The root word "phleb" pertains to veins. For example, "phlebitis" refers to inflammation of a vein.

- What does the prefix "syn-" mean?
  Answer: Together or with - The prefix "syn-" indicates together or with. For example, "synergy" refers to the interaction of elements that produce a combined effect greater than the sum of their individual effects.

- What does the suffix "-scope" mean?
  Answer: Instrument for viewing - The suffix "-scope" denotes an instrument for viewing. For example, "microscope" refers to an instrument used to view small objects.

- What does the root word "thorac" refer to?
  Answer: Chest - The root word "thorac" pertains to the chest. For example, "thoracotomy" refers to a surgical incision into the chest wall.

- What does the prefix "retro-" mean?
  Answer: Backward or behind - The prefix "retro-" indicates backward or behind. For example, "retrograde" refers to moving backward.

- What does the suffix "-tomy" mean?
  Answer: Cutting or incision - The suffix "-tomy" denotes cutting or incision. For example, "tracheotomy" refers to an incision into the trachea.

EXTRA CONTENTS

Audiobook

We are pleased to offer an additional bonus: a complimentary audiobook version. This allows you to reinforce your learning through audio.

400+ Digital Flashcard

These digital flashcards have been designed to consolidate your knowledge and help you.

3 Playlist Video | 52 VIDEO

With these 3 Playlists you can learn by watching videos.

https://medicalterminologymadeeasy.newpublishingagency.com/step-1-page-2176-8651-9785

Made in the USA
Las Vegas, NV
18 October 2024

96936399R00096